H. Devlin
Operative Dentistry

Hugh Devlin

Operative Dentistry

A Practical Guide to Recent Innovations

With 75 Figures in 102 Separate Illustrations and 5 Tables

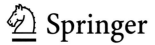
Springer

Dr. Hugh Devlin
School of Dentistry
The University of Manchester
Higher Cambridge Street
Manchester
M15 6FH
United Kingdom

Library of Congress Control Number: 2005939045

ISBN-10 3-540-29616-6 Springer Berlin Heidelberg New York
ISBN-13 978-3-540-29616-4 Springer Berlin Heidelberg New York

This work is subject to copyright. All rights reserved, whether the whole or part of the material is concerned, specifically the rights of translation, reprinting, reuse of illustrations, recitation, broadcasting, reproduction on microfilm or in any other way, and storage in data banks. Duplication of this publication or parts thereof is permitted only under the provisions of the German Copyright Law of September 9, 1965, in its current version, and permission for use must always be obtained from Springer. Violations are liable for prosecution under the German Copyright Law.

Springer is a part of Springer Science+Business Media
springer.com
© Springer-Verlag Berlin Heidelberg 2006
Printed in Germany

The use of general descriptive names, registered names, trademarks, etc. in this publication does not imply, even in the absence of a specific statement, that such names are exempt from the relevant protective laws and regulations and therefore free for general use.

Product liability: The publishers cannot guarantee the accuracy of any information about dosage and application contained in this book. In every individual case the user must check such information by consulting the relevant literature.

Editor: Gabriele Schröder, Heidelberg
Desk Editor: Martina Himberger, Heidelberg
Cover design: Frido Steinen-Broo, eStudio Calamar, Spain
Typesetting and production: LE-TEX Jelonek, Schmidt & Vöckler GbR, Leipzig, Germany
Printed on acid-free paper   24/3100/YL - 5 4 3 2 1 0

Preface

This book embraces the most recent developments in modern operative dentistry, but has attempted to merge these with traditional practice. Students, colleagues, and general dental practitioners have requested an evidence-based approach to the practical concepts in modern restorative dentistry. One important philosophy that is emphasized in this book is that the prevention of dental caries, restoration failure, and periodontal disease should be the basis of all operative dentistry. Recent developments in restoration design and material science technology are also assessed in the light of the best available evidence, which is referred to in the text. Innovative instrument design is described and useful practical techniques are explained.

The worldwide use of amalgam will continue to decline as patients demand better aesthetic restorations. For this reason, posterior resin-composite restorations, ceramic inlay/onlay restorations, and the new high-strength porcelain crown systems are given considerable prominence in this book. The new adhesive technologies are especially useful in the treatment of tooth erosion that may have resulted from the consumption of carbonated beverages.

This is a medium-sized textbook that should be used in conjunction with larger reference texts, journal reviews, and other publications. It should complement other books in the field and will hopefully stimulate further reading.

I am indebted to my friends and colleagues who generously provided illustrations. Dr. David Reekie provided the photograph in Fig. 2.15, Dr. Catherine Potter provided those in Figs. 2.4 and 2.5, Dr. Ian Pretty provided those in Figs. 1.5–1.7, and Dr. Peter Geertsema, whose excellent standard of dental treatment is acknowledged throughout Europe, provided all of the photographs in Figs. 5.11–5.14. Their generous assistance is gratefully acknowledged.

Contents

1	**New Methods of Detection of Caries**	1
1.1	The Diagnosis of Caries	1
1.1.1	DIAGNOdent	5
1.1.2	Digital Imaging Fiber-Optic Transillumination	7
1.1.3	Fiber-Optic Transillumination	8
1.1.4	Quantitative Light-Induced Fluorescence	9
1.1.5	Radiology of Dental Caries	10
1.1.6	Electrical Conductance	12
1.1.7	Modern Caries Detection and Management	12
	References	13
2	**New Developments in Caries Removal and Restoration**	17
2.1	Caries Removal	17
2.1.1	Lasers	18
2.1.2	Polymer Bur	20
2.1.3	Micropreparation Burs	20
2.1.4	Air Abrasion (or Kinetic Cavity Preparation)	21
2.1.5	Photoactivated Disinfection	23
2.1.6	Carisolv Gel	23
2.1.7	Atraumatic Restorative Treatment	24
2.1.8	Caries-Detector Dyes	25
2.2	Restoration Following Caries Detection	26
2.2.1	Why Are Teeth Restored?	26
2.2.2	Caries as a Disease	27
2.2.3	Preventing Dental Caries	28
2.2.4	When Should Caries Be Restored?	30
2.2.5	Fissure Sealants	32
2.2.6	Ozone Therapy for the Treatment of Caries	32
2.3	Restorative Procedures	34
2.3.1	The "Tunnel" Restoration	34
2.3.2	The Proximal "Slot" Preparation	34
2.3.3	Traditional Cavity Preparation	35

2.3.4	The Repaired Amalgam Restoration	37
2.3.5	Cavity Preparations Involving Three or More Surfaces	37
2.3.6	Treatment of the Large Carious Lesion	38
2.3.7	The Use of Calcium Hydroxide in Direct Pulp Capping	40
2.3.8	The Foundation Restoration	41
2.3.9	Practical Aspects of Amalgam Retention	42
2.3.10	Pins vs Bonded Restorations	43
2.3.11	Amalgam Bonding Procedure	44
2.3.12	The Use of Base Materials	45
	References	45
3	**Posterior Resin Composite Restorations**	51
3.1	Ramped Curing Lights	52
3.2	Ceramic Inserts	52
3.3	Nanotechnology	54
3.4	"Total Etch" Technique	54
3.5	Fissure Sealants	55
3.6	Preventive Resin Restorations	56
3.7	Minimal Class II Restorations	57
3.8	Posterior Composite Resin Restoration	57
3.9	Direct Composite Resin Restorations	58
3.10	Studies of Direct Resin-Composite Restoration Survival	60
3.11	Reasons for Failure of Extensive Direct Composite Resin Restorations	60
3.12	The "Sandwich" Technique	62
3.13	Packable Composite Resin Materials	62
3.14	New Developments in Resin-Composite Technology	64
	References	64
4	**The Single Crown, Veneers, and Bleaching**	67
4.1	The Single Crown	67
4.1.1	Recurrent Caries and Periodontal Disease	67
4.1.2	The Tooth Becomes Nonvital	69
4.1.3	The Crown Restoration Becomes Loose	69
4.1.4	Perforation of the Crown During Occlusal Adjustment	73
4.1.5	The Appearance of the Crown is Unsatisfactory	74
4.1.5.1	Shade of the Crown	75
4.1.5.2	Shape of the Crown	76
4.1.5.3	Gingival Contour	76
4.1.5.4	Gingival Recession	76
4.2	New Developments in Crown Provision	78

4.3	Veneers	79
4.3.1	Tooth Preparation	79
4.3.2	Disadvantages of Veneers	81
4.3.3	Failure of Veneers	81
4.3.4	Cementation Procedures for a Veneer	83
4.3.5	Provisional Restorations for Veneers	83
4.4	Resin-Bonded All-Ceramic Crowns (or "Dentin-Bonded Crown")	84
4.4.1	Marginal Leakage	86
4.4.2	Cementation Procedures for the Resin-Bonded All-Ceramic Crown	86
4.5	Bleaching of Teeth	87
4.5.1	Cervical Resorption	87
4.5.2	The "Walking Bleach" Technique	88
4.5.3	Vital Tooth Bleaching	89
4.5.4	In-House Tooth Bleaching	90
4.6	Microabrasion	90
	References	92
5	**Noncarious Tooth Tissue Loss**	95
5.1	Noncarious Tooth Wear	95
5.1.1	Clinical Appearance of Erosion	95
5.1.2	Clinical Appearance of Attrition	96
5.1.3	Clinical Appearance of Abrasion	97
5.2	Prevention of Toothwear	97
5.3	Recent Developments in the Treatment of Tooth Wear	100
5.3.1	Noncarious Cervical Restorations	100
5.3.2	Clinical Procedures for Restoration of Cervical Lesions	100
5.3.3	Why Do Cervical Restorations Fail?	101
5.3.4	New Developments in Direct Posterior Resin Composites	103
5.3.5	Addition of Resin Composite to Anterior Teeth	104
5.3.6	Developments in Indirect Resin Composite Technology	105
5.3.6.1	Targis/Vectris Crowns	106
5.3.6.2	Sinfony	106
5.3.6.3	Belleglass HP	106
5.3.6.4	Other Fiber Systems	107
5.4	Ceramic Inlay and Onlay Restorations	107
5.5	Inlay Restorations	108
5.6	Onlay Restorations	109
5.6.1	Milled Ceramic Inlays or Onlays	111
5.6.1.1	Cerec 3	111

5.6.1.2	IPS Empress System	112
5.6.1.3	Fortress	113
5.7	Full-Veneer Posterior Porcelain Crowns	115
5.7.1	In-Ceram	115
5.7.2	Procera AllCeram Crowns	116
5.8	Cementation of the Restoration	117
5.9	Choosing the Correct Restorative System	118
5.10	Conclusion	119
	References	119

Subject Index 123

1 New Methods of Detection of Caries

1.1
The Diagnosis of Caries

Simply looking at a tooth to determine whether caries is present is an inaccurate technique, although the exact sensitivity and specificity depends upon the experience of the dentist (Huysmans et al. 1998). The diagnosis of caries is one of the most difficult clinical assessments that the dentist must perform (Fig. 1.1a,b). For the best results, the teeth should be dried, and when good illumination is used a carious occlusal lesion affecting the outer half of the enamel will appear white and opaque. The anatomy of the occlusal fissure is often invaginated to form an expanded hidden chamber that is easily colonized by bacteria and then can become carious. However, when the walls of the fissure have incipient caries, the lesion is easily missed by the examining dentist. Where the occlusal demineralization progresses to affect the outer third of the dentin, an obvious white-spot lesion is visible without drying the surface. Frank cavitation of the enamel surface occurs usually when the inner half of the dentin has undergone demineralization and is accompanied by softening of the outer dentin (Ekstrand et al. 1998). When cavitation of the tooth surface occurs, plaque removal by the patient becomes impossible and progression of the lesion is inevitable. Caries progresses further by spreading along the enamel-dentin junction and undermining the overlying enamel (Fig. 1.2). Caries is a dynamic process that involves alternating periods of dissolution of tooth mineral and its reformation, depending on the acidity of the plaque environment. A radiopaque band is often seen pulpal to the carious lesion and results from the reprecipitation of calcium and phosphate previously dissolved by the carious process.

Due to the reprecipitation of calcium and phosphate, the hardness of carious dentin increases to a maximum at a point a few millimeters away from the soft surface dentin This is seen if a carious tooth is sectioned and hardness measurements are made at intervals from the carious surface to the normal, unaffected dentin (Fig. 1.3). In the experiment shown in Fig. 1.3, the

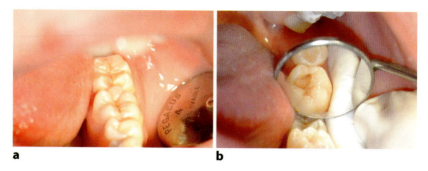

Fig. 1.1 (a) Caries is one of the most difficult diseases to diagnose. (b) Deep dentinal caries beneath an intact enamel surface can often be invisible to the examining dentist

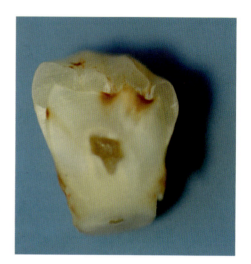

Fig. 1.2 Caries undermines enamel by spreading laterally along the dentinoenamel junction, resulting in a cone-shape dentinal lesion

hardness of the teeth was tested at loads of 100 mN and 500 mN. The surface zone of soft dentinal caries has undergone proteolysis, whereas the underlying couple of millimeters of dentin have undergone demineralization and varying degrees of proteolysis. Caries progresses by alternate demineralization (when the pH falls) and subsequent partial remineralization by regrowth of apatite crystals (when the pH rises). The reprecipitation of calcium and phosphate ions at the demineralization front often produces a radiopaque zone. For the remaining zone of demineralized dentin, calcium and phosphate ions are lost as they diffuse away into saliva. The surface dentin is destroyed by proteolytic enzymes and can be easily removed with hand instruments. Between the surface and the radiopaque band there is a demineralized zone,

1.1 The Diagnosis of Caries

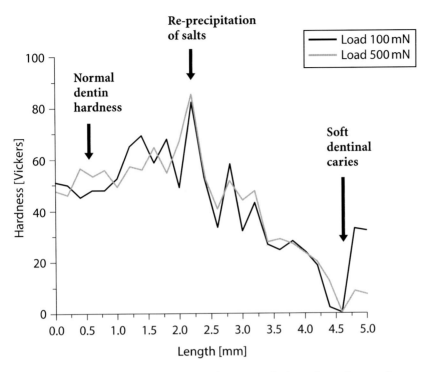

Fig. 1.3 Hardness measurements recorded at intervals from the carious surface to the normal unaffected dentin. Moving away from the softened carious dentin, there is a gradual increase in hardness, so that at 2 mm hardness has returned to that of normal dentin

which contains no bacteria and should be preserved during tooth preparation. As can be seen from Fig. 1.3, the hardness of demineralized carious dentin in the 1-mm zone adjacent to the reprecipitation zone may be only slightly less than that of normal, unaffected dentin.

If the enamel overhanging a carious cavity is removed, the carious process will often arrest, and the dentin surface becomes hard and dark brown in color (Fig. 1.4). However, color is unreliable as a method of distinguishing active from inactive lesions. The patient rarely complains of symptoms because a protective layer of tertiary dentin is formed at the pulpal end of the dentinal tubule. This provides an impermeable barrier because the dentinal tubules of tertiary dentin are not in continuity with those of the overlying primary or secondary dentin.

Radiographs also have their limitations in diagnosing caries, but fortunately there have been recent technological developments in caries diagnosis.

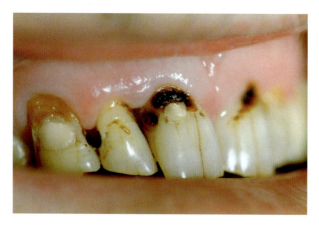

Fig. 1.4 In the elderly, there is an increased incidence of carious lesions affecting the cervical margins. This may result from multifactorial causes such as a change in diet, sugary medicines, declining health, xerostomia, and gingival recession

Radiographs cannot detect occlusal carious lesions that are confined to enamel (Ekstrand et al. 1997), because the width of the unaffected enamel obscures any effect of the demineralized carious lesion. The sensitivity of a caries detection system measures how good a test is at detecting caries when it is truly present. Specificity measures how good a test is at detecting the absence of caries when there is truly no caries present. In general, bitewing radiography has poor sensitivity and specificity for minimal occlusal caries detection (Attrill and Asley 2001), but is better than visual inspection alone. Radiography taken on one occasion is unable to distinguish an actively progressing from a passive lesion, or a cavitated from a noncavitated surface. Deep dentinal lesions that are visible on a radiograph are more likely to be cavitated. Demineralized, noncavitated lesions may be arrested, but the main body of the demineralized, dentin usually remains radiolucent.

Progressive mineral loss in a carious lesion can be detected between successive radiographic films by digitally subtracting the information on one film from that on the other, provided similar projection angles are used. Unchanged areas are conventionally displayed in a gray color, whereas areas of mineral loss appear a darker gray. There have been successful laboratory studies, but the technique remains experimental.

Dentists in general dental practice report that most of their restorations are replaced because of secondary caries (Mjor and Toffenetti 2000), although this is a vague diagnosis. Secondary caries is a lesion at the margin of an existing restoration and should be distinguished from ditching and staining around the amalgam filling. Small marginal defects, crevices, and ditches do not give rise to secondary caries. The grayish-stained enamel and dentin often seen with secondary caries must be distinguished from the staining that arises from diffusion of amalgam into the surrounding tooth substance, or staining around the margin of a restoration associated with microleakage. Staining around the margin of a restoration is not a reliable predictor of the presence of carious dentine beneath it (Kidd et al. 1994). Unfortunately, visual indicators are poor indicators of the necessity for operative intervention, as only a clearly visible carious lesion is predictive of underlying dentinal caries. Sensitivity measures the proportion of true positives (i.e., the proportion of carious cavities that are correctly diagnosed), and is low for the diagnosis of occlusal caries by visual inspection.

Use of a probe to detect caries can damage teeth and cavitate lesions that might otherwise remineralize. Using a probe to "stick" into the fissure to detect fissure caries is unreliable and therefore should be abandoned. Penning et al. (1992) examined 100 extracted teeth with stained fissures and found that use of a probe to detect carious lesions had low sensitivity (i.e., only 22% of the carious lesions were revealed by probing). If a fine, pointed probe is used then it is possible to diagnose caries where none exists (poor specificity). This is because the probe becomes wedged in the healthy fissure. Probing for suspected lesions can cause cavitation of lesions that were previously limited to the subsurface of enamel (van Dorp et al. 1988).

1.1.1
DIAGNOdent

There are other recent developments in caries detection that have improved sensitivity and specificity over visual diagnosis. DIAGNOdent

(Kavo, Biberach/Riß) uses a pulsed red light (655 nm wavelength) to illuminate the tooth (Fig. 1.5a) and analyses the emitted fluorescence from bacterial products (Fig. 1.5b), which changes with tooth demineralization. The demineralization is given a numerical value that relates to the fluorescence intensity. This technique can be used for the accurate diagnosis of primary occlusal caries and caries on flat, accessible surfaces (Bamzahim et al. 2004), but it does not detect interproximal or subgingival caries. Where the dentist has instituted preventive measures for the demineralized enamel lesion, this technique provides an objective method of assessment of lesion progression. DIAGNOdent may be a useful technique to monitor a patient's readings from visit to visit and enables the dentist to provide feedback to them about the progress of their preventive regime. However, a consistent methodology must be used for successive measurements as there is some variation in measure-

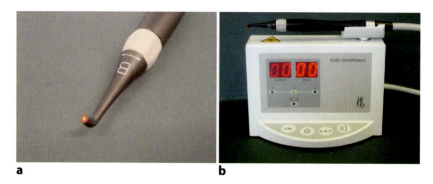

Fig. 1.5 (a) The DIAGNOdent probe emits a red light, which is shone onto the tooth. (b) DIAGNOdent: The emitted fluorescence from the tooth surface changes with tooth demineralization

ment depending upon dehydration of the tooth and whether or not plaque is present (Mendes et al. 2004). The manufacturers recommend that the teeth be cleaned prior to taking any readings, although DIAGNOdent readings are increased by polishing teeth with a pumice paste. The appropriate probe is chosen, and after calibration the probe is moved over the occlusal fissures, rotating buccolingually as it is moved in the mesiodistal direction. Dependent on the caries risk of a patient and other diagnostic information, DIAGNOdent readings between 5 and 20 indicate preventive therapy, with sealants used when the readings are between 10 and 30. Readings above 30 indicate active caries removal.

Lussi et al. (1999) found that DIAGNOdent had a sensitivity of 0.76–0.84 and a specificity of 0.79–0.87 in the detection of dentinal caries on the occlusal surface. Shi et al. (2000) found that DIAGNOdent was significantly better than radiography at detecting occlusal caries. Using a value above 18–22 as diagnostic of a carious lesion, they found that DIAGNOdent had a good sensitivity of 0.78–0.82 in detecting carious dentin. However, they reported that the instrument could give erroneous readings with stain, plaque, and calculus, as well as areas of developmental hypoplasia or hypomineralization. The in vitro studies by Shi et al. (2000) and Lussi et al. (1999) may not be applicable to the clinical situation as they used teeth with a high prevalence of caries and the disinfectant solutions used to store the teeth may have been far more effective at removing plaque than could be achieved clinically in the office by the dentist.

Some studies have concluded that the agreement between the extent of validated caries and the laser fluorescence value is still unsatisfactory (Heinrich-

Weltzien et al. 2003). A study by Iwami et al. (2004) found that the lowest DIAGNOdent value at which bacteria were detected in dentin was 15.6, with no bacteria detectable at readings lower than this. This would indicate that the DIAGNOdent reading relates to the degree of bacterial infection. However, insufficient data exist to recommend that DIAGNOdent be used as a method of indicating to the dentist how deep he should excavate caries. This is because the diameter of the DIAGNOdent tip is large, so gaining access to the exact location of the carious dentin in the cavity is unclear. The DIAGNOdent device has been shown to give a wide range of readings for enamel caries (7–100), superficial dentinal caries (7–100), and deep dentinal caries (12–100). The device is therefore unable to distinguish between superficial and deep dentinal caries, probably because the laser light is unable to reach the deep dentin (Lussi et al. 2001). The wide overlap of readings makes this an unreliable method of measuring the depth of dentin caries.

Composite restorative materials emit fluorescence and amalgam emits none, so the diagnosis of secondary caries under these restorative materials is unreliable, despite claims that caries under clear fissure sealants can be detected. Hosoya et al. (2004) showed that following the application of sealants, the DIAGNOdent values recorded were reduced. Visual examination has a high specificity in caries diagnosis and is rapid. The role of a device such as DIAGNOdent may be to provide corroboratory evidence of caries or to investigate a fissure of diagnostic uncertainty. DIAGNOdent is a useful technique in diagnosing caries, provided there is adherence to the recommended protocol. DIAGNOdent is more sensitive than visual methods at detecting caries, but there is also an increased likelihood of a false-positive diagnosis (Bader and Shugars 2004). In the future, DIAGNOdent, used with fluorescent dyes, may prove useful in delineating cavitated from noncavitated approximal carious lesions.

1.1.2
Digital Imaging Fiber-Optic Transillumination

Digital imaging fiber-optic transillumination (DIFOTI, Electro-Optical Sciences, Irvington, USA) uses visible light, not ionizing radiation, and is approved by the US Food and Drug Administration for the detection of caries on approximal, smooth, and occlusal surfaces, as well as recurrent caries. DIFOTI uses the scattering of light by carious tissue as a method of distinguishing it from healthy enamel, therefore subgingival lesions cannot be visualized using this system. Light is passed through the tooth, collected using a camera, and the image displayed on a computer screen. The system has a choice of mouthpieces. The interproximal mouthpiece (detecting interproximal caries) shines light from either the buccal or lingual surface, which is imaged on the opposite side by a CCD camera in the handpiece. The occlusal mouthpiece (detecting occlusal caries) gathers light originating from the buccal and lingual tooth surface. In both cases, a standard personal computer with an image capture card allows the image to be viewed on a monitor.

The carious part of the tooth appears dark against a light background of the healthy tooth. Image acquisition is fast as there is no processing time involved. Light may be scattered by hypomineralized enamel and deeply stained fissures, which may therefore be difficult to distinguish from carious lesions. Prior prophylaxis of the tooth with a powder jet may go some way toward reducing this problem. Unfortunately, the dentist is given no information of lesion depth relative to the enamel-dentin junction, so it may be difficult to monitor the progression of a lesion if a preventive program is instituted. There is no computer assistance in diagnosis; the dentist must decide if caries is present.

Schneiderman et al. (1997) found that the DIFOTI technique has superior sensitivity over conventional radiological methods for the detection of approximal, occlusal, and smooth-surface caries, and specificity was slightly less in general. DIFOTI is therefore able to detect early surface carious lesions not readily discernible by radiographic film technology. The greater sensitivity of DIFOTI may mean that white-spot carious lesions with an intact enamel surface may appear dark and be erroneously diagnosed as requiring restoration. The value of this technique may be to encourage a preventive approach by patients as they can readily visualize the demineralized enamel. Other studies support the use of fiber-optic transillumination (FOTI, see 1.1.3) and DIFOTI in the diagnosis of occlusal caries. Fennis-Ie et al. (1998) found that 44% of the sites diagnosed as having enamel or dentinal caries by FOTI actually became carious within 2.5 years. The DIFOTI technique is rapid, and images are instantly available following capture by the dentist. These images can then be discussed with the patient.

1.1.3
Fiber-Optic Transillumination

The FOTI technique has been reported as a useful adjunct to clinical caries examination and a useful diagnostic tool in general dental practice (Davies et al. 2001). FOTI is as accurate as a detailed visual inspection in detecting occlusal caries (Cortes et al. 2000). Unfortunately, FOTI has a low sensitivity in detecting interproximal caries (Vaarkamp et al. 2000).

1.1.4
Quantitative Light-Induced Fluorescence

The quantitative light-induced fluorescence (QLF) system (Fig. 1.6; manufactured by Inspektor Research Systems, Amsterdam, The Netherlands) uses a blue light (~488 nm wavelength) to illuminate the tooth, which normally fluoresces a green color. Teeth should be dried for 15 s to produce more consistent readings (Pretty et al. 2004). Carious lesions appear as dark areas. The reflected light is passed through a yellow filter, and after processing is displayed in real time on a computer monitor. A decrease in fluorescence is associated with tooth demineralization and lesion severity. Images can be captured and analyzed to provide measurements of lesion area, lesion depth, and lesion volume. This information is very useful for monitoring enamel lesions on a longitudinal basis to see how they respond to a preventive regime. The technique does not use ionizing radiation and is completely safe. However, QLF will only detect enamel demineralization and cannot distinguish between caries limited to the enamel and that which extends into dentin (Tam and McComb 2001). The depth of the carious lesion in dentin cannot be related to the intensity of the fluorescence (Bannerjee and Boyd 1998). In addition, QLF cannot distinguish between decay and hypoplasia. Despite this, the QLF technique has a high sensitivity and specificity in detecting caries that has progressed into dentin. Haftröm-Björkman et al. (1991) found a sensitivity of 0.72–0.76 and a specificity of 0.79–0.81 for this technique.

QLF can also be used to image plaque and calculus, and may therefore be useful in identifying active caries. This useful technique has found many applications in clinical trials, research, patient education, and preventive clinical

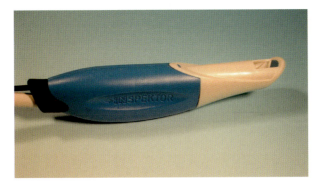

Fig. 1.6 The quantitative light-induced fluorescence system (QLF system, Inspektor Research Systems, Amsterdam, The Netherlands)

practice. The technique can effectively monitor demineralization and remineralization of teeth in vitro, and a good correlation has been reported with other techniques measuring mineral loss, such as transverse microradiography analysis (Pretty et al. 2003b). QLF has also been used to assess the erosive potential of a range of mouthwashes in vitro, and shown that they pose little danger in this respect (Pretty et al. 2003a). Several studies have now shown that QLF can be used successfully to detect early secondary caries around amalgam and tooth-colored filling materials (Gonzalez-Cabezas et al. 2003). Demineralization of enamel adjacent to orthodontic brackets is an unfortunate complication of orthodontic treatment, especially if it is not detected early and remedial action take. QLF can be used to detect enamel demineralization and the success of a subsequent fluoride remineralization regime (Pretty et al. 2003c).

1.1.5
Radiology of Dental Caries

The caries process causes demineralization of teeth, which is evident as a radiolucency of the affected tissues. Radiological diagnosis is particularly valuable in the identification of interproximal caries and recurrent caries, whereas other diagnostic methods may be less accurate. Good-quality radiographic caries diagnosis requires a bitewing projection and beam-aiming device to minimize overlap of the teeth. This intraoral technique is superior to panoramic radiography (Scarfe et al. 1994). A comparison of the sensitivity and specificity of radiographic and visual examinations is given in Table 1.1.

Occlusal caries confined to enamel is not identifiable on radiographs because of the substantial thickness of overlying, sound enamel, which prevents adequate contrast. Occlusal caries has to be quite advanced in dentin before enamel radiolucency and cavitation are seen on the radiograph. Radiography

Table 1.1 Mean sensitivity and specificity associated with radiographic and visual detection of cavitated carious lesions (Bader et al. 2001)

Technique	Sensitivity of detection	Specificity of detection
Visual		
Occlusal lesions	63	89
Proximal lesions	94	92
Radiography		
Proximal lesions	66	95

is extremely useful in diagnosing interproximal caries, which occurs between the contact point of adjacent teeth and the gingival crest. The triangular-shaped enamel lesion has a base at the surface and the apex pointing toward the enamel-dentin junction. When the interproximal caries progresses to reach the enamel-dentin junction, it spreads laterally to form a triangular-shaped dentinal lesion, which then extends toward the pulp. On radiograph, the base of the triangular carious dentin lesion lies on the enamel-dentin junction and the apex points toward the pulp.

The critical issue in assessing whether to intervene and restore a carious tooth is whether the carious lesion has cavitated. Of lesions confined to the inner enamel, about half have been shown by visual inspection to be cavitated, but this is not easy to detect radiographically. Instead, the depth of the carious lesion is usually used as an indicator of cavitation and hence of restorative intervention. Cavitation occurs in about 70% of carious lesions that appear to be confined radiographically to the outer dentin. Enamel and dentin lesions have a true depth that is greater than the radiological lesion depth, because approximately 40% of the mineral has to be removed before this is visible radiographically. Given this uncertainty, it is not surprising that there is a wide disparity among dentists concerning restorative treatment thresholds for approximal surfaces and in opinions about the rate of caries progression (Tubert-Jeannin et al. 2004).

False-positive radiological diagnoses of caries occur with cervical "burn-out" and the "Mach band" effect. Cervical burnout is an artifact that occurs as a result of the X-ray beam passing through only a thin edge of dentin at the neck of the tooth. The beam is attenuated very little and the region appears radiolucent. Cervical burnout extends to the alveolar bone crest, which distinguishes it from interproximal caries. Burnout is increased where the exposure is greater and where contrast is high with an overlying metallic crown restoration. The "Mach band" effect is an illusion that results from viewing two areas of differing optical density, such as enamel and dentin. A dark line is perceived on the dentinal surface and caries may be incorrectly diagnosed (a false positive). This dark "Mach band" effect is usually limited to a line 0.5 mm below the enamel-dentin junction.

Whether the newer methods of caries detection replace the routine use of regular bitewing radiographs is not known, but there is increasing public concern about the use of ionizing radiation in a low caries prevalent population.

1.1.6
Electrical Conductance

This method uses the increase in electrical conductivity of a tooth when it is demineralized. Conductivity is measured from the enamel surface to a ground electrode, and any increase in conductivity is due to microscopic demineralized spaces within the enamel. Several studies have used electrical conductance measurement to detect caries, employing equipment such as the Electronic Caries Monitor (ECM; Lode Diagnostic, Groningen, The Netherlands). This is a battery-powered device that has an alternating current output with a low frequency of approximately 21 Hz (Fig. 1.7a,b).

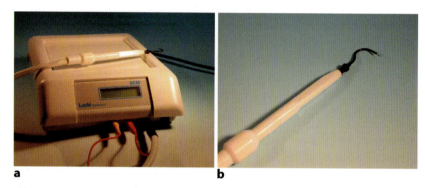

Fig. 1.7 (a) Electronic Caries Monitor (ECM, Lode Diagnostic, Groningen, The Netherlands). (b) The ECM has an excellent sensitivity in detecting occlusal caries, but its specificity is lower. It may have less reproducibility than other caries-detecting systems such as DIAGNOdent

Some studies have found the ECM technique to be less reproducible than other measurement systems (such as DIAGNOdent). This may be due to the variation in conductance caused by surface moisture producing differences in conductance between the ECM probe and the tooth (Ellwood and Cortes 2004), or to varying degrees of dehydration of the tooth. Despite this, ECM has an impressive sensitivity (93%) in detecting occlusal caries, with an overall accuracy of 83%; however, its specificity remains relatively low at 77% (Lussi et al. 1995).

1.1.7
Modern Caries Detection and Management

Caries is difficult to diagnose with 100% accuracy, but the minimum investigation should include a visual examination with bitewing radiographs. This fact alone should encourage the dentist to be cautious in restoring teeth in a population with low caries risk. Modern caries management suggests that lesions should not be restored unless there is frank cavitation present or until the radiolucency has extended into the outer third of interproximal dentin. This means that there is no indication for restoring stained fissures, where no dentinal radiolucency exists. Techniques that provide an objective assessment of the presence of caries (such as electrical conductance, DIAGNOdent, or computer analysis of radiographs) have an advantage over techniques such as DIFOTI and conventional radiography, which require interpretation by the dentist.

The opposite opinion is often expressed, that the earliest interception of decay maintains dental health and a "wait and see" philosophy is neglectful. Boyd et al. (1952) studied a population of children with learning difficulties and, despite their poor oral hygiene, found that the median length of time for mild dentinal involvement to take place was about 3 years. A proportion of incipient carious lesions will not progress and will remineralize, but assessing whether a lesion is remineralizing or progressing to decay is difficult. In those patients attending regularly, the risk of missing caries is lower than the risk of unnecessary treatment.

If ultraconservative interventionist treatments are carried out at the earliest stage of caries development, then the opportunity for remineralization to take place is not permitted. Where all diagnostic methods are inconclusive as to whether a stained fissure is indeed carious, exploration of the fissure with a small round, or a very fine short tapered bur can be used to obtain a definitive diagnosis. This can then be restored in an ultraconservative manner.

The clinician must, of course, assess the potential for caries in a cavity based on a visual examination of the tooth, the patient's history, and radiographs, but be aware of the limitations of all diagnostic devices. The correct treatment appropriate for each patient must depend upon their caries risk, co-operation with diet advice, dental, social, and medical history, and no single, blanket treatment philosophy will be appropriate for all patients.

References

Attrill DC, Ashley PF. Occlusal caries detection in primary teeth: a comparison of DIAGNOdent with conventional methods. Br Dent J 2001; 190:440–443.

Bader JD, Shugars DA. A systematic review of the performance of a laser fluorescence device for detecting caries. J Am Dent Assoc 2004; 135:1413–1426.

Bader JD, Shugars DA, Bonito AJ. Systemic reviews of selected dental caries diagnostic and management methods. J Dent Educ 2001; 65:960–968.

Bamzahim M, Shi XQ, Angmar-Månsson B. Secondary caries detection by DIAGNOdent and radiography: a comparative in vitro study. Acta Odontol Scand 2004; 62:61–64.

Bannerjee A, Boyd A. Autofluorescence and mineral content of carious dentine: scanning optical and backscattered electron microscopic studies. Caries Res 1998; 32:219–226.

Boyd JD, Wessels KE, Leighton RE. Epidemiologic studies in dental caries. J Dent Res 1952; 31:124–128.

Cortes DF, Ekstrand KR, Elias-Boneta AR, Ellwood RP. An in vitro comparison of the ability of fibre-optic transillumination, visual inspection and radiographs to detect occlusal caries and evaluate lesion depth. Caries Res 2000; 34:443–447.

Davies GM, Worthington HV, Clarkson JE, Thomas P, Davies RM. The use of fibre-optic transillumination in general dental practice. Br Dent J 2001; 191:145–147.

Ekstrand KR, Rickets DN, Kidd EA. Reproducibility and accuracy of three methods for assessment of demineralization depth of the occlusal surface: an in vitro examination. Caries Res 1997; 31:224–231.

Ekstrand KR, Ricketts DN, Kidd EA. Do occlusal carious lesions spread laterally at the enamel-dentin junction? A histolopathological study. Clin Oral Investig 1998; 2:15–20.

Ellwood RP, Cortes DF. In vitro assessment of methods of applying the electrical caries monitor for the detection of occlusal caries. Caries Res 2004; 38:45–53.

Fennis-Ie YL, Verdibschot EH, van't Hof MA. Performance of some diagnostic systems in the prediction of occlusal caries in permanent molars in 6- and 11-year-old children. J Dent 1998; 26:403–408.

Gonzalez-Cabezas C, Fontana M, Gomes-Moosbauer D, Stookey GK. Early detection of secondary caries using quantitative, light-induced fluorescence. Oper Dent 2003; 28:415–422.

Hafström-Björkman U, Sundström F, Angmar-Månsson B. Initial caries diagnosis in rat molars, using laser fluorescence. Acta Odontol Scand 1991; 49:27–33.

Heinrich-Weltzien R, Kuhnisch J, Oehme T, Ziehe A, Stosser L, Garcia-Godoy F. Comparison of different DIAGNOdent cut-off limits for in vivo detection of occlusal caries. Oper Dent 2003; 28:672–680.

Hosoya Y, Matsuzaka K, Inoue T, Marshall GW Jr. Influence of tooth-polishing pastes and sealants on DIAGNOdent values. Quintessence Int 2004; 35:605–611.

Huysmans MC, Longbottom C, Pitts NB. Electrical methods in occlusal caries diagnosis: an in vitro comparison with visual inspection and bite-wing radiography. Caries Res 1998; 32:324–329.

Iwami Y, Shimizu A, Narimatsu M, Hayashi M, Takeshige F, Ebisu S. Relationship between bacterial infection and evaluation using a laser fluorescence device, DIAGNOdent. Eur J Oral Sci 2004; 112:419–423.

Kidd EA, Joyston-Bechal S, Beighton D. Diagnosis of secondary caries: a laboratory study. Br Dent J 1994; 176:135–138, 139.

Lussi A, Firestone A, Schoenberg V, Hotz P, Stich H. In vivo diagnosis of fissure caries using a new electrical resistance monitor. Caries Res 1995; 19:81–87.

Lussi A, Imwinkelried S, Pitts N, Longbottom C, Reich E. Performance and reproducibility of a laser fluorescence system for detection of occlusal caries in vitro. Caries Res 1999; 33:261–266.

References

Lussi A, Megert B, Longbottom C, Reich E, Francescut P. Clinical performance of a laser fluorescence device for detection of occlusal caries lesions. Eur J Oral Sci 2001; 109:14–19.

Mendes FM, Hissadomi M, Imparato JC. Effects of drying time and the presence of plaque on the in vitro performance of laser fluorescence in occlusal caries of primary teeth. Caries Res 2004; 38:104–108.

Mjor IA, Toffenetti F. Secondary caries: a literature review with case reports. Quintessence Int 2000; 31:165–179.

Penning C, van Amerongen JP, Seef RE, ten Cate JM. Validity of probing for fissure caries diagnosis. Caries Res 1992; 26:445–449.

Pretty IA, Edgar WM, Higham SM. The erosive potential of commercially available mouthrinses on enamel as measured by Quantitative Light-induced Fluorescence (QLF). J Dent 2003a; 31:313–319.

Pretty IA, Edgar WM, Higham SM. The effect of dehydration on quantitative light-induced fluorescence analysis of early enamel demineralization. Oral Rehabil 2004; 31:179–184.

Pretty IA, Ingram GS, Agalamanyi EA, Edgar WM, Higham SM. The use of fluorescein-enhanced quantitative light-induced fluorescence to monitor de- and re-mineralization of in vitro root caries. J Oral Rehabil 2003b; 30:1151–1156.

Pretty IA, Pender N, Edgar WM, Higham SM. The in vitro detection of early enamel de- and re-mineralization adjacent to bonded orthodontic cleats using quantitative light-induced fluorescence. Eur J Orthod 2003c; 25:217–223.

Scarfe WC, Langlais RP, Nummikoski P, Dove SB, McDavid WD, Deahl ST, Yuan CH. Clinical comparison of two panoramic modalities and posterior bite-wing radiography in the detection of proximal dental caries. Oral Surg Oral Med Oral Pathol 1994; 77:195–207.

Schneiderman A, Elbaum M, Shultz T, Keem S, Greenebaum M, Driller J. Assessment of dental caries with Digital Imaging Fiber-Optic TransIllumination (DIFOTI): in vitro study. Caries Res 1997; 31:103–110.

Shi XQ, Welander U, Angmar-Månsson B. Occlusal caries detection with KaVo DIAGNOdent and radiography: an in vitro comparison. Caries Res 2000; 34:151–158.

Tam LE, McComb D. Diagnosis of occlusal caries: Part II. Recent diagnostic technologies. J Can Dent Assoc 2001; 67:459–463.

Tubert-Jeannin S, Domejean-Orliaguet S, Riordan PJ, Espelid I, Tveit AB. Restorative treatment strategies reported by French university teachers. J Dent Educ 2004; 68:1096–1103.

Vaarkamp J, ten Bosch JJ, Verdonschot EH, Bronkhoorst EM. The real performance of bitewing radiography and fiber-optic transillumination in approximal caries diagnosis. J Dent Res 2000; 79:1747–1751.

van Dorp CS, Exterkate RA, ten Cate JM. The effect of dental probing on subsequent enamel demineralization. ASDC J Dent Child 1988; 55:343–347.

2 New Developments in Caries Removal and Restoration

2.1
Caries Removal

There have been several recent developments with regard to methods of caries removal, and new laser, air abrasion, and chemomechanical methods have been introduced, as well as improvements in the more traditional bur technology. Laser and air-abrasion machine technologies do not contact the tooth, and as such they are much less likely than the traditional dental bur to become contaminated and cause cross-infection. Single-use dental burs prevent cross-infection, but their cost can be prohibitive. Cleaning dental burs using only autoclaving does not result in satisfactory decontamination, and a presterilization cleaning must be implemented. Manual cleaning of burs with a bur brush may produce a variable quality of presterilization cleaning, is laborious and time-consuming, and support staff may suffer puncture wounds of their skin. Washer disinfectors are very effective for presterilization cleaning of contaminated burs (Whitworth et al. 2004), but these machines are costly. Ultrasonic cleaners used with enzymatic detergents (at 60 °C) have been shown to completely kill all *Streptococcus mutans* in suspensions after 20 min of sonication (Bettner et al. 1998).

Traditional methods of caries removal, such as burs and spoon excavators, tend to remove uninfected as well as infected dentin, because it is difficult clinically to distinguish between the two. However, total removal of all caries may not be necessary to control progression of the lesion, provided the restoration is sealed adequately from the oral environment. The harder surface of inner caries can form a hybrid layer with adhesive resin, the bond strength of which is not as high as that of normal dentin, but forms an adequate sealed restoration. Recent developments in caries removal have therefore involved removal of only soft infected dentin.

2.1.1
Lasers

Early use of infrared lasers, such as carbon dioxide (10.6 μm wavelength) and ruby lasers, to remove carious dentin resulted in slow removal of tissue and excessive heat transfer to the dental pulp. Lasers have achieved success with removal of hyperplastic soft tissue, but sufficient research has now established the use of other laser technologies in restorative dentistry.

Traditional removal of carious dentin with a bur does involve some discomfort. One of the main advantages of lasers is the absence of vibration, which alleviates much of the discomfort experienced by patients. Despite the precision of lasers, the absence of tactile contact with the tooth during cavity preparation can make detection of softened dentin difficult for the dentist. The erbium yttrium aluminum garnet (erbium:YAG, 2.94 μm wavelength) laser has received much research interest, and in 1997, the Food and Drug Administration approved the erbium:YAG laser for caries removal in the USA. The Fidelis erbium:YAG laser (Fotona, Ljubljana, Slovenia) is one example of the commercially available lasers for dental use, but it is a rather large device (Fig. 2.1), with settings for varying the cutting speed (Fig. 2.2).

Erbium:YAG laser treatment of teeth produces no smear layer, so the adaptation of filling materials to the enamel and dentin surfaces should be optimal.

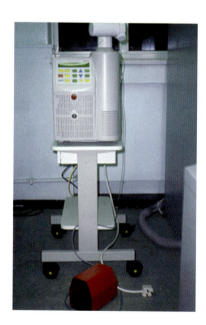

Fig. 2.1 The erbium-YAG laser is commercially available, but many perceive it as costly and offering few advantages over conventional methods of cavity preparation. The machine is large and occupies considerable space in the dental office

2.1 Caries Removal

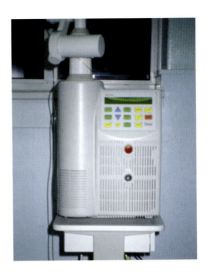

Fig. 2.2 The erbium:YAG laser can safely remove dentin and enamel in a cavity preparation provided water cooling and optimal laser parameters are used. Adjustment of the laser cutting speed is possible

This might be expected to improve the adaptation and retention of adhesively retained resin composites to the tooth. However, experimental results with the erbium:YAG laser have been disappointing (Eguro et al. 2002), probably because laser irradiation weakens the surrounding dentin. Erbium:YAG preparation of enamel must be followed by conventional etching with phosphoric acid if adequate adhesion of resin composites to enamel is to be achieved (Otsuki et al. 2002).

The erbium:YAG laser energy ablates tissues by being absorbed by water, causing a rapid rise in temperature and pressure, and resulting in a microexplosion of dentin and enamel. The dentinal tubules are therefore left open. The degree of thermal damage experienced by the pulp is difficult to assess because most of the studies have been performed on extracted teeth. Hoke et al. (1990) embedded thermal probes into the pulp chambers of extracted teeth during cavity preparation with an erbium:YAG laser and water mist, and found an average rise in temperature of only 2.2 °C. A water mist prevents a high rise in temperature, washes away ablated tissue, and improves the rate of ablation. However, much higher and shorter-duration temperature increases must be present in dental tissues closer to the laser beam, and these are much more difficult to detect. Dostalova et al. (1997) used an erbium:YAG laser to prepare cavities in human premolar teeth prior to extraction, and found no evidence of inflammation of the pulp or cracking in the dentin. The evidence would suggest that the erbium:YAG laser can safely remove dentin and enamel in a cavity preparation provided water cooling and optimal laser parameters are used.

Dentists perceive the erbium:YAG laser at its present stage of development as offering few advantages over conventional methods of cavity preparation (Dederich and Bushick 2004; Evans et al. 2000). The main advantage is that lasers are noiseless, which nervous patients find helpful. However, focusing of the erbium:YAG laser beam is difficult due to pooling of the water spray on the tooth surface, and this defocusing effect results in a marked reduction in ablation efficiency. Preparing undercut surfaces is not possible as tissue can only be removed when it is visible in the operator's line of sight.

Further developments in laser technology are possible with lasers having femtosecond pulse duration (Kohns et al. 1997), but these are still in the highly experimental stages and are not ready for clinical dental application (Fig. 2.3).

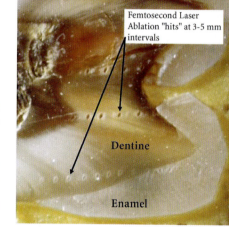

Fig. 2.3 These holes were created by a femtosecond laser (laser pulse duration = 10^{-15} s). The femtosecond laser can photoablate bone, enamel, and dentine with the minimum of collateral thermal damage. This laser is still in the experimental stage of development for dental use

2.1.2
Polymer Bur

Boston (2000) has described a polymer bur that only removed softened and infected dentin and not normal dentin. The cutting elements of the bur were made of a softer polyamide/imide polymer material than the traditional carbide bur.

2.1.3
Micropreparation Burs

The Fissurotomy Bur (SS White Burs, Lakewood, NJ, USA) is designed to allow exploration of the fissure with minimal removal of enamel. It is 1.5–2.5 mm in length and tapers to a fine carbide tip so that only one-sixth to one-tenth of the intercuspal width is removed. Other burs such as the Brassler 889M-007 bur (Brasseler USA, Savannah, GA, USA) allow minimally invasive preparation of the tooth occlusal surface, and where slightly wider preparation is required, the Micro-Diamond 838M-007 can be used.

Microinstruments (such as the Micropreparation set 4337, by Brasseler, Germany) require low contact pressure (< 2 N) to avoid instrument breakage. The instruments are manufactured using special high-tensile steel, producing a thin neck.

2.1.4
Air Abrasion (or Kinetic Cavity Preparation)

This technique uses a stream of small aluminum oxide particles, created using pressurized air, that impact the caries and abrade it away. However, the abrasive particles tend to remove normal dentin more easily than the softer, carious dentin. One of the main advantages of the air abrasion technique is that there is less pain associated with cavity preparation than with conventional bur preparation, perhaps because there is less noise and vibration. Malmstrom et al. (2003) found that all ten subjects in their study preferred air abrasion over conventional rotary bur preparation for removing fissural caries. Most of their subjects experienced no pain with this minimal tooth preparation. Rafique et al. (2003) also showed that a substantial majority (75%) of their patients were unperturbed by any dust or pain sensation during cavity preparation.

Air abrasion of enamel does not provide enough micromechanical roughening of enamel for the retention of composite resins (Jahn et al. 1999). Having prepared a tooth cavity using air abrasion, the enamel must be treated with acid-etchant in the conventional way for satisfactory retention of a composite resin. There is little tactile sensation when removing softened carious dentin as the instrument does not touch the tooth, so the indications for use of this instrument tend to be limited to minimal cavity preparation and the removal of surface enamel stain.

Figure 2.4 shows a typical air-abrasion system (Prep Start, Danville Engineering San Ramon, California, USA). The variable pressure settings and powder flow rates (27-µm or 50-µm diameter alumina particles) ensure that treatment of minor caries lesions can be treated in an ultraconservative manner. The handpiece is light (Fig. 2.5) and the flow of powder (0.7 – 4.2 g/min) has a continuously controlled variable outflow.

Air polishing devices use sodium bicarbonate powder, and can remove plaque and stain effectively. These devices cause no harm to the gingiva,

Fig. 2.4 Air abrasion systems allow minimal cavity preparation and the removal of surface stain

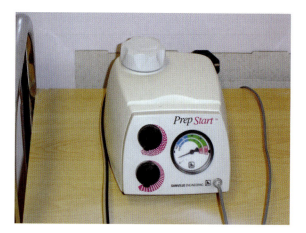

Fig. 2.5 The air abrasion handpiece is light and the flow of powder has a controlled variable outflow

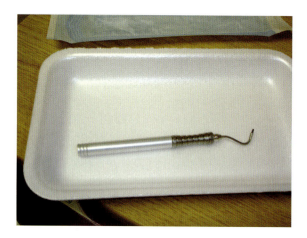

but they have the disadvantage that they can easily cause iatrogenic damage by removing exposed cementum and root dentin in teeth affected by gingival recession and periodontal disease. Atkinson et al. (1984) found that their air-powder abrasive system removed a mean depth of 637 µm of root structure in 30 s of exposure time. Further research aimed at identifying less abrasive powders is ongoing (Petersilka et al. 2003), because softer particles might be more effective in removing carious dentin more selectively. Laurell et al. (1995) showed in dogs that higher pressures and smaller particles yielded significantly fewer pulpal effects than treatment with high-speed rotary burs.

2.1.5
Photoactivated Disinfection

The photoactivated disinfection technique (Denfotex Light Systems, Inverkeithing, UK) uses a disinfectant solution that is applied to deep caries, allowed to penetrate into the remaining softened dentin for 60 s, and then photoactivated for 1 min using a low-powered diode laser (635 nm). The disinfectant solution is dilute toluidine blue, which binds to the bacteria in the carious lesion. Activation with the red light releases oxygen, which kills the cells. The tooth is restored using an adhesively retained restoration. The laser light penetrates well into the softened dentin and adjacent healthy tissues are not damaged by heat or applied chemicals. Toluidine blue is safe at the dilution used (the LD50 of toluidine blue is 10 mg/kg; 95% confidence interval 7.35–13.60 mg/kg; Cudd et al. 1996).

A solution of toluidine blue activated using laser light energy (at 633 nm) has been shown to kill *S. mutans* (Williams et al. 2003). Neither the laser nor the toluidine blue solution was effective when used alone, but when used together they were very effective.

Further clinical trials are required to determine whether this technique has advantages over cheaper techniques such as simply applying calcium hydroxide to the softened dentin to encourage remineralization.

2.1.6
Carisolv Gel

Carisolv (MediTeam Dental, Göteborgsvägen, Sweden) is a chemomechanical method of removing dental caries that is minimally invasive. First of all a fluid is mixed consisting of a cocktail of amino acids and 0.5% sodium hypochlorite, and is applied to the dentin. The amino acids and hypochlorite form high-pH chloramines (pH 12), which react with the denatured collagen in the carious dentin, allowing it to be removed more easily. The softened dentin is removed by scraping the surface with special hand instruments.

This technique requires longer clinic time than similar cavity preparation employing conventional bur removal (Kavvadia et al. 2004). However, because only soft carious dentin is affected and not normal dentin, the need for anesthesia is reduced (Kakaboura et al. 2003), which is a major advantage in dental-phobic patients, children, and special needs patients. The technique is useful for the removal of root or coronal caries where access is easily obtained, but requires repeated application of the solution over the caries. Use of Carisolv Gel may be an inefficient method of removing caries at the enamel-dentin junction. Carious dentin may go unnoticed beneath the overhanging enamel because ideal access may require extensive preparation with a rotary bur (Yazici et al. 2003). However, in this region, conventional removal of caries with a bur can be demanding, even when using magnifying loops. Kidd et al. (1989) showed that demineralized dentin remained at the enamel-dentin junction in 57% of cavities that had originally been assessed as caries-free using conventional visual and tactile means. Some bacteria will remain at the enamel-dentin junction whatever approach is adopted (Kidd 2004), therefore stained, hard dentin should be left alone in this area and no attempt should be made to remove it. Carisolv Gel removes the smear layer and has no adverse effect on the bond strength of adhesive materials to dentin.

Should Carisolv come into contact with exposed pulp tissue, no toxic effect should be expected. Young et al. (2001) found no adverse effects with Carisolv when it was left in contact with rat pulp tissue. Bulut et al. (2004) exposed the pulp chambers of 40 human first premolars with class V cavities and applied either Carisolv or sterile saline solution for 10 min. The cavities were restored with a compomer filling material and the teeth extracted after either 1 week or 1 month. No adverse histologic effects due to Carisolv were observed.

2.1.7
Atraumatic Restorative Treatment

The atraumatic restorative treatment (ART) technique was first introduced in rural areas of developing countries. The soft caries is removed with hand instruments and the cavity restored with a glass ionomer restoration. Critics of the technique state that bacteria are left in the hand-excavated cavities, which is certainly true, but the total amount of bacteria is much reduced (Bonecker et al. 2003). In clinical field studies, restorations performed using this approach tend to wear and fail as a result of loss of the glass ionomer, but have a much reduced rate of secondary caries compared with amalgam restorations (Mandari et al. 2003). High wear of the glass ionomer after 30 months was also reported by Gao et al. (2003) in their hospital clinic study.

There is a great, unmet need for dental treatment among the increasing numbers of elderly in industrialized countries. ART would seem to be a cost-effective method of providing treatment for these patients in their home or protected environment. The technique does not usually require anesthetic and produces little discomfort for the patients. In a Finnish study, Honkala and Honkala (2002) placed 33 ART restorations and evaluated 25 of them 1 year later. Four of the restorations were graded as having an unacceptable marginal defect, and one filling was totally lost. This was a short-term study, but they concluded that this was an acceptable survival rate of restorations.

The bond strength of glass ionomer to caries-affected dentin is much less than the bond strength of the more modern resin-modified glass ionomer (Palma-Dibb et al. 2003). The additional resin content makes the latter materials stronger and more esthetic, as well as providing fluoride release. In addition, the wear of traditional glass ionomer restorations means that the patients require frequent review by trained dental health personnel. Some have called for ART restorations to be confined to single-surface carious lesions, given the relatively high rate of failure of glass ionomer restorations (Smales and Yip 2002). Single-surface ART restorations have a survival rate similar to that of amalgam restorations over 3 years (Frencken et al. 2004).

2.1.8
Caries-Detector Dyes

Modern management of caries involves removing infected dentin, but in as conservative a manner as possible to preserve tooth tissue. In this way, the weakening of tooth structure is prevented, pulp vitality preserved, and the treatment cycle of increasingly more extensive restorations is avoided. In caries removal during cavity preparation, only the soft, heavily infected outer dentin must be removed, whereas the demineralized, uninfected inner dentin should be left. Caries-detecting dyes (e.g., 1.0% acid red in propylene glycol) have been developed to assist the dentist in distinguishing between the two types of caries (Fusayama 1988).

Clinically, the method is simple to perform. The suspected carious lesion is first washed with water and dried with an air syringe. One drop of a solution of caries-detecting dye is applied to the dentin surface for 10 s, and then washed off and dried. High-volume aspiration is essential to prevent the dye being either swallowed or ejected out of the mouth onto clothing. The dyes stain infected carious dentin (Fig. 2.6), but also stain the demineralized organic matrix of carious dentin, and are therefore limited in their usefulness. Areas of carious-free teeth that have a naturally lower mineral content (e.g., circumpulpal dentine and the enamel-dentine junction) are also stained (Yip et al. 1994). Using caries-detecting dyes as the sole criteria for tooth substance removal has been shown to result in gross overpreparation of the carious cavity (Banerjee et al. 2003), but caries-detecting dyes may be a useful adjunct in assisting the clinician to assess caries (Thomas et al. 2000). Preventing the ingress of bacterial nutrient from the oral cavity by sealing the carious dentin would anyway arrest a small amount of undiagnosed dentinal caries.

Caries-detecting dyes have no place in the detection of occlusal fissure caries, primarily because these dyes stain the normal dentin at the enamel-dentin junction (Kidd et al. 1989). False-positive diagnoses are also likely

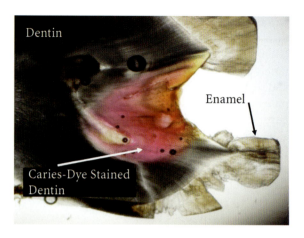

Fig. 2.6 Caries-detecting dyes stain infected carious dentin, but also stain the demineralized organic matrix of carious dentin, which should not be removed. Their use will result in overpreparation of the tooth, therefore they are not recommended

because these dyes will stain food debris and other organic material in the fissure. The consequences of a false-negative diagnosis (i.e., the dentist concluding that fissure caries is absent when it is truly present) are less significant than providing an unnecessary restoration.

2.2 Restoration Following Caries Detection

2.2.1 Why Are Teeth Restored?

Unfortunately, restorations in general dental practice survive on average for about 7 years (Burke et al. 2001), which is much less time than they should. According to one review, one in three of all restorations present at any one time is unsatisfactory (Elderton 1976a). The reasons for operative intervention given by dentists in various studies include primary caries, secondary caries, marginal fracture, and noncarious defects. When teeth enter the restorative cycle, subsequent replacement inevitably results in weakening of the tooth, cusp replacement and increasingly complex restorations with further increased potential for failure. To obtain maximum longevity for a restoration, the dentist must use skill, well-tried techniques and products, and encourage the patient to maintain good oral hygiene. At least half of all restorations placed in the dental office are replacements of existing restorations. The main reasons for failure of a restoration are: (1) excessive occlusal loading (e.g., due to a nonworking side interference), (2) errors in cavity design (e.g., lack of retentive undercut), (3) poor choice of restorative material, and (4) poor management of the gingival tissues (e.g., encroachment of the restoration onto the epithelial or connective tissue attachment; the "biological width").

As the incidence of caries is declining in the developed world and as dental materials improve in quality, the need for traditional invasive treatment will decline and be replaced by a modern, preventive approach.

2.2.2
Caries as a Disease

Caries is a transmissible, infectious disease, and the risk of future caries must be eliminated before definitive restorative treatment begins. The acidogenic bacteria are *S. mutans* and lactobacilli, and elevated numbers of these bacteria in saliva ($> 10^5$ cfu/ml *S. mutans* and $> 10^3$ cfu/ml lactobacilli) are indicative of high caries activity. A certain salivary concentration of *S. mutans* is required for colonization of occlusal fissures of teeth. All patients should have a caries risk assessment based on their previous caries experience, medical history, use of fluoride in water or toothpaste, and an oral examination. Exposed root surfaces, a poor quality of tooth restoration or poorly designed denture, carious lesions, and tooth crowding can all contribute to a high caries risk. Other indicators of high caries risk include frequent sugar intake, xerostomia, radiation therapy, Sjogren's syndrome, self-abusive behavior (e.g., drug addiction or alcoholism), and poor manual dexterity resulting in poor oral hygiene. Figure 2.7 illustrates the reduced, deteriorating dentition of a patient with poor oral hygiene. Commercially available test kits are available to test the saliva consistency, quality, pH, and buffering capacity (e.g., GC Saliva Check, Newport Pagnell, UK; Fig. 2.8). Universal indicator paper will change to a green color in saliva with a neutral pH (Fig. 2.9).

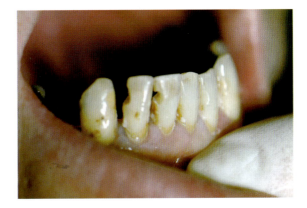

Fig. 2.7 Oral hygiene instruction and diet advice are essential to prevent further deterioration of this dentition

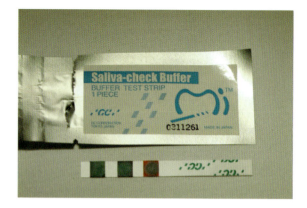

Fig. 2.8 Commercially available test kits are available to test saliva consistency, quality, pH, and buffering capacity

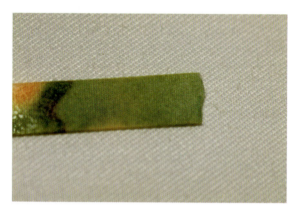

Fig. 2.9 Universal indicator paper can provide a visual indication to the patient of their salivary pH. The lime green color illustrated indicates a normal salivary pH

2.2.3 Preventing Dental Caries

When combined with the reduction in the consumption of frequent fermentable carbohydrate, a regime consisting of a once daily rinse of 0.05% fluoride mouthwash is effective in arresting or reversing the progression of early enamel lesions. Mouthwashes consisting of 0.12% chlorhexidine are available and can be used twice daily for 3 weeks. Chlorhexidine is an effective antimicrobial treatment for caries and periodontal disease, but causes a brown stain to form on the teeth if used routinely. Many manufacturers have available mouthwashes, sprays, and gels containing fluoride, and minerals such as calcium and phosphate.

Patients at high risk of caries (Fig. 2.10) should have a course of 0.12% chlorhexidine mouthwash (Peridex, Zila) followed by at-home daily 0.05%

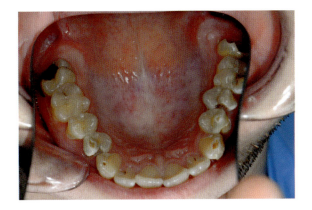

Fig. 2.10 Extensive caries is now seldom seen in the general population, because of the widespread use of fluoridated toothpaste combined with patients' increasing expectation of good oral health. Rampant caries is still seen in disadvantaged groups such as drug addicts

fluoride mouthwash. In-office fluoride gel applications are also helpful. They consist of applying 2% neutral sodium fluoride gel for 4 min every week for 4 weeks. This regime can be repeated every 6 months. The dentist can apply small quantities of fluoride varnish (fluoride at a concentration of 22,600 ppm in a resin base) directly to an early noncavitated lesion. Fluoride varnish (Duraphat, Colgate; Fluor Protector, Vivadent), when applied to the decalcified enamel lesion, will encourage remineralization. The teeth are dried and isolated from saliva with cotton wool rolls and when the varnish is applied it adheres to the enamel. Chlorhexidine causes unsightly brown staining of the teeth if used persistently (Fig. 2.11). The stain may require professional removal with prophylaxis paste.

High-caries-risk patients require regular clinical and microbiological examinations every 3–6 months. The microbiological assay test can be used to

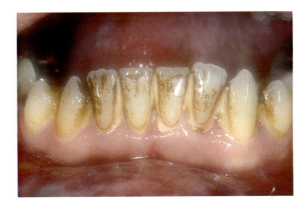

Fig. 2.11 Chlorhexidine causes an unsightly brown staining of the teeth if used persistently

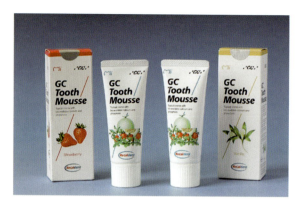

Fig. 2.12 Mineral-rich pastes are available that can be used to remineralize the tooth. These pastes are pleasant tasting and have no side effects

confirm that the chlorhexidine has been effective in bacterial suppression. Xylitol chewing gum has also been shown to be effective and its use is recommended three times a day after meals; it stimulates salivary flow, which will tend to buffer acid in plaque and assist in enamel remineralization. GC Tooth Mousse is a new, water-based, topical cream containing Recaldent casein phosphopeptide–amorphous calcium phosphate. When applied to the tooth surface, calcium phosphate is made available for remineralization of the tooth surface. The mineral-rich paste has a pleasant taste, which should stimulate salivary flow (Fig. 2.12).

All patients should receive instruction on how to maintain their dentition plaque free and be advised to use fluoridated toothpaste twice a day. Normal brushing cannot remove all plaque from the fissures of teeth, so oral hygiene status does not have any definitive relationship with the prevalence of fissure caries. Reduction of the frequency of sugar intake is extremely important in preventing further decay. Dietary counseling should reduce the frequency of cariogenic foods (especially sucrose) and also suggest other carbohydrate substitutes.

2.2.4
When Should Caries Be Restored?

Preventive care is advised even for those large lesions that are progressive and/or are cavitated because the etiological factors must be removed if the caries is to be eliminated in the long term. A restorative and preventive approach must both be used. Cavitated lesions cannot be cleaned of accumulating plaque and their continuous progression is inevitable, so they should be restored. In noncavitated lesions, bacterial infection is usually absent. Determining whether the surface of a carious enamel lesion has broken can be difficult to recognize in approximal dental caries. Radiographs do not provide this information.

Foster (1998) concluded that lesions extending deeper than 0.5 mm into the dentin on radiograph should be considered for restoration. He found that 92% of lesions extending over 0.5 mm and up to 1 mm into dentin progressed further over 3 years, whereas only 50% of more shallow lesions extending 0.5 mm into dentin progressed in the same way. Whether a lesion progresses depends primarily upon whether the lesion has cavitated. Lesions that are confined to enamel have a low probability of being cavitated, and therefore a preventive approach should be adopted. Pitts and Rimmer (1992) found that lesions, which on radiograph appear to extend to the outer half of dentin, have a 41% chance of being cavitated, whereas radiolucencies that extend to the inner half of dentin were always cavitated. It is commonly stated that all lesions that appear on radiograph to involve dentin should be restored, because the caries will have spread further clinically than is evident on the radiograph. However, of those lesions that involve the outer dentin, less than half are cavitated and this would result in an erroneous restoration of these teeth on about half (59%) of occasions. The caries risk of the patient will influence whether an interventive or preventive approach is instituted, because the probability of progression of the lesion must be affected by their overall caries risk.

If it is to be successful, the preventive approach requires a significant change in a patient's consumption of sucrose, and should include a reduction in the frequency and amount of cariogenic foods and carbohydrate substitution. This requires a change in a patient's lifestyle and is not easily achieved. Hintze et al. (1999) studied approximal lesions visible on radiograph in the outer

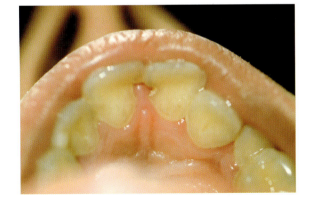

Fig. 2.13 An open, cavitated carious lesion may cause chronic irritation of the adjacent gingiva resulting in gingival hypertrophy. The excess tissue should be cauterized prior to restoring the cavity

dentin and reported that even amongst well-motivated dental students, 20% of the lesions cavitated within an 18-month period.

Sometimes an open, cavitated, carious lesion will cause mechanical irritation of the adjacent gingiva (Fig. 2.13). Gingival hypertrophy into the open cavity then ensues. Satisfactory restoration of this cavity will require prior cautery of the hyperplastic gingival tissue.

2.2.5
Fissure Sealants

Resin composite materials are sensitive to moisture, and have a reduced success rate in erupting molars where good isolation is difficult. Even though teeth appear clinically to be well sealed, nearly 50% have marginal defects on scanning electron microscopy (Fig. 2.14).

But, where fissure sealants have been placed over carious lesions for several years, predominantly negative bacterial cultures are recorded (Going et al. 1978; Handelman et al. 1976). However, GC Fuji VII (GC Europe, Belgium) is a glass ionomer that adheres to enamel and dentin in the presence of moisture. It is a translucent, pink-colored material that can be placed over the fissure surface, and does not require prior etching of the enamel.

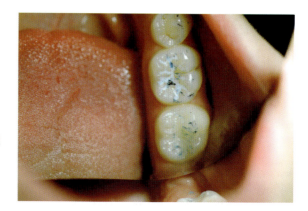

Fig. 2.14 Fissure sealants should be used in recently erupted teeth, when the tooth is most vulnerable to caries

2.2.6
Ozone Therapy for the Treatment of Caries

Dental caries is caused by bacteria, and as ozone will kill certain bacteria, many studies have investigated whether ozone is effective in arresting the progression of caries. No serious side effects to the treatment have been reported.

2.2 Restoration Following Caries Detection

Advocates of this treatment modality recommend ozone as a disinfectant gas to eliminate bacteria from occlusal caries (up to 2 mm in depth), root carious lesions, and pit and fissure lesions, often with the absence of further operative treatment. The carious lesion is encouraged to remineralize over 4 weeks using fluoride and mineral mouthwashes, toothpaste, and sprays. Baysan and Lynch (2004) found that ozone application for 10–20 s eliminated most of the microorganisms found in primary root caries lesions. Ozone can reduce the numbers of *S. mutans* and *S. sobrinus* on saliva-coated glass beads in vitro (Baysan et al. 2000). However, the role that this disinfection process can play in the long-term reversal of previously active carious lesions is controversial. Rickard et al. (2004) analyzed the available published literature and concluded that "given the high risk of bias in the available studies and lack of consistency between different outcome measures, there is no reliable evidence that application of ozone gas to the surface of decayed teeth stops or reverses the decay process." Further research is necessary.

With the HealOzone system (KaVo Dental, Biberach, Germany), ozone gas is delivered via a special handpiece that fits over and bathes the tooth (Fig. 2.15).

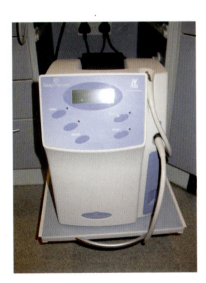

Fig. 2.15 HealOzone (KaVo Dental, Biberach, Germany) delivers ozone gas, which disinfects the tooth. The minimally carious lesion is encouraged to remineralize over a period of 4 weeks using fluoride and mineral mouthwashes, toothpaste, and sprays

2.3
Restorative Procedures

2.3.1
The "Tunnel" Restoration

The approximal caries is removed by gaining access from the occlusal surface and preserving the marginal ridge. The caries is removed and the enamel on the approximal surface smoothed. Most of the clinical studies report using silver-cermet glass ionomer as the preferred restorative material. This technique has fallen from favor because of the difficulty of completely removing the caries, subsequent frequent collapse of the marginal ridge, and occlusal wear of the restorative material. Hasselrot (1998) reported a 50% survival rate of tunnel restorations in permanent teeth over a 6-year period.

2.3.2
The Proximal "Slot" Preparation

In the "slot" preparation, access to the caries is gained through the marginal ridge, but preserving this structure wherever possible (Mount and Ngo 2000). The occlusal fissure is maintained intact and when the cavity is restored with resin-composite, the fissure can be protected with sealant. The cavity design allows better visualization of the caries than the tunnel design, allowing the removal of unsupported enamel. The cavity can be restored with glass ionomer and a bonded surface laminate of composite resin to resist heavy occlusal contact (Fig. 2.16).

Slot preparations to be restored with amalgam require mechanical retention. Grooves 0.5-mm wide must be cut into the facial and lingual walls of the

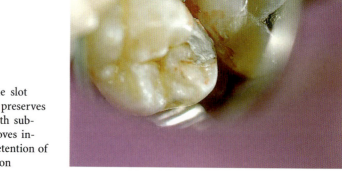

Fig. 2.16 The slot preparation preserves occlusal tooth substance. Grooves increase the retention of the restoration

proximal box using the full diameter of a No1/4 round bur. They are placed 0.25 mm from the enamel-dentin junction in the opposing facial and lingual walls, and parallel to the external surface of the tooth. The grooves should be quite distinct, extending from the gingival floor of the slot preparation to the occlusal surface.

2.3.3
Traditional Cavity Preparation

There seems a great deal of confusion in the literature as to what constitutes success and failure in treatment where amalgam restorations have been provided. To the dentist confronted with a patient's failed amalgam it would seem essential that he/she diagnose the reason for the failure so that the same failure does not recur in the new restoration. Many studies have used vague criteria for clinical failure with little objectivity, yet a great deal of time and money is devoted to replacing existing amalgam restorations. Elderton and Davis (1984) found that two-thirds of all restorations in Scotland were replacements of existing restorations.

Major causes of operative treatment failure include secondary caries and bulk fracture of the amalgam (Jokstad and Mjör 1991). Bulk fracture at the occlusal isthmus of a class II cavity preparation is a common cause of restoration failure (Fig. 2.17) and may be due to a sharp axiopulpal line angle, insufficient bulk of amalgam, or excessive thickness of a weak cement lining (Fig. 2.18). Others have associated the creation of amalgam edge angles of less than 70° and poor adaptation of the amalgam to the cavity margin as indicating a failed restoration (Elderton 1976b). Marginal defects in amalgam restorations are poor indicators of whether recurrent caries is present (Merret and Elderton

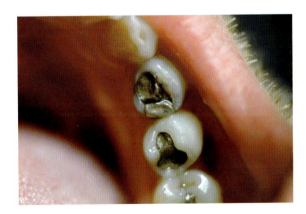

Fig. 2.17 Bulk fracture of the amalgam at the occlusal isthmus region is a common reason for failure of these restorations

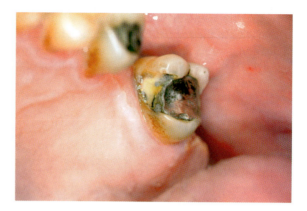

Fig. 2.18 Excessively thick base cement has resulted in an insufficient thickness of amalgam. The resulting restoration was severely weakened and fracture inevitable

1984). Whether recurrent caries is associated with marginal amalgam defects often depends upon the overall caries risk of the patient (Goldberg et al. 1981). So in considering whether to replace the deficient restoration shown in Fig. 2.19, the overall caries risk of the patient must be assessed. Whereas features such as a gingival overhang of the restoration margin certainly reduce the quality of the resulting restoration, opinion is divided as to whether even such a restoration should be replaced (Paterson et al. 1995). Similarly, there is disagreement among experts about the need for operative intervention where white spots or dentinal staining exist adjacent to restoration margins (Paterson et al. 1995). However, most would agree that the loss of an amalgam restoration or its fracture should require replacement or repair to prevent secondary caries.

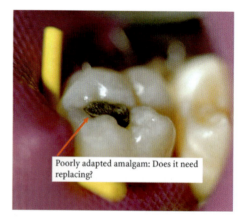

Fig. 2.19 Better clinical guidance about when to replace restorations is required, but an important factor for the dentist to consider is the overall caries risk of the patient

2.3.4
The Repaired Amalgam Restoration

Repairing a fractured amalgam restoration would seem a cost-effective method of treatment in many cases. In addition, the size of a repaired restoration can often be kept smaller than if the whole of the original restoration was replaced. Cipriano et al. (1995) examined 45 repaired restorations over a 2-year period and found that 98% of these restorations had acceptable junctions between the old and new amalgam. No secondary caries was found. Other studies have found similar high rates of success. Smales and Hawthorne (2004) found that after 5 years, repaired amalgams had survived as well as replaced amalgams. Van Nieuwenhuysen et al. (2003) found a success rate of 82% in all types of repaired restorations. Using resin bonding agents does not significantly increase the bond strength of amalgam to amalgam (Nuckles et al. 1994). McDaniel et al. (2000) found that amongst cuspal coverage amalgam restorations, the main cause of failed restoration was fracture of the restoration as the main reason, followed by secondary caries and tooth fracture. Cusps are weakened when their height exceeds the width of their base; therefore reduction of the height of weak cusps is necessary to allow cuspal coverage of amalgam. Adequate resistance form usually requires a reduction of 1.5 mm on the nonsupporting cusp and 2 mm on the supporting cusp.

The distobuccal cusp of the lower first molar is often weakened, despite preparation of a conservative distal box. A conservative preparation will involve breaking contact with the adjacent second molar to provide a space of 0.5 mm. This may weaken the distobuccal cusp of the first molar to occlusal forces, requiring it to be reduced by 1.5 mm for coverage by amalgam.

2.3.5
Cavity Preparations Involving Three or More Surfaces

Cavities involving preparation of the mesial, occlusal, and distal surfaces inevitably weaken the tooth and therefore require special attention to minimal removal of tooth tissue. Cuspal reduction and coverage is indicated if the facial or lingual extension of the occlusal cavity exceeds two thirds the cusp height. The reduced cuspal height should allow an amalgam restoration of 2 mm occlusal height.

Provided the oblique ridge of the maxillary first molar is not undermined, it should be preserved and caries on the mesial and distal surfaces restored separately. In the same way, the mandibular first molar has a transverse ridge, which, if preserved, can give strength to the tooth. The proximal lesions are then restored separately.

2.3.6
Treatment of the Large Carious Lesion

Before treatment can be undertaken, the patient's symptoms must be elicited together with a detailed clinical examination. The patient may report pain of short duration (10 s or less) following a cold stimulus, which would indicate a reversible pulpitis. The pulp would be expected to maintain vitality and the pain to disappear when the caries has been removed and the tooth restored. If the pain from the tooth should last longer than 10 s with a cold stimulus, then an irreversible pulpitis is indicated.

A clinical examination will utilize electrical and thermal pulp testing of the carious tooth and adjacent neighboring teeth, measurement of periodontal pocket depths, and occlusal analysis. The extent of the breakdown of the tooth is noted, as well as any swelling or sinus openings in the buccal sulcus. Traditional treatment of the large carious lesion has involved using calcium hydroxide to either cover a pulpal exposure (direct pulp cap) or cover the softened dentin with a view to stimulating the formation of reparative dentin (indirect pulp cap). Figure 2.20 illustrates the coverage of a near pulpal exposure by calcium hydroxide.

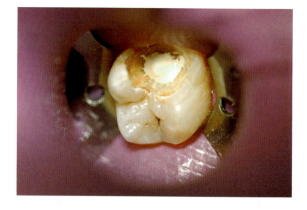

Fig. 2.20 Calcium hydroxide cement has poor strength and is soluble, but is still the preferred material to place on the dentinal floor of very deep cavities

The success of direct pulp capping, measured in terms of an absence of symptoms, and maintenance of pulpal vitality and blood supply (Ricketts 2001) is increased where: (1) the pulp is pink and any hemorrhage is easily controlled by washing with sterile saline, (2) there is a normal vital response, (3) there is no radiographic pathology, (4) there is no previous spontaneous pain, (5) the tooth has no tenderness to percussion, and (6) the patient is young and where the pulp would be expected to be more vascular than in an older individual. However, the sealing of the cavity to prevent microleakage is absolutely critical to the success of direct pulp capping. Studies that have used only a zinc oxide eugenol restorative material have shown a poor success rate. Efficiently sealing the cavity may have much more influence on the success rate of direct pulp capping than other factors such as the chronological age of the pulp (Mestrener et al. 2003). Figure 2.21 shows a pulp exposure that was treated successfully by covering with calcium hydroxide and sealing with an adhesive restoration.

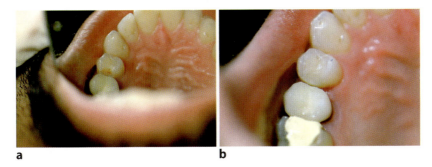

Fig. 2.21 (a) This was a small pulpal exposure in the upper premolar tooth, but little bleeding was evident. The tooth was isolated from salivary contamination, and calcium hydroxide applied to the exposure. (b) With the calcium hydroxide placed over the pulpal exposure, a coronal seal was established with a glass ionomer base and adhesively retained composite resin restoration. The tooth remained vital and symptomless

With direct pulp capping, the size of a traumatic pulpal exposure is irrelevant to the likely success of treatment (Klein et al. 1985). Some recommend the surface removal of 2 mm of the pulp to eliminate dentinal debris (a potent source of pulpal inflammation), followed by disinfection of the pulp cavity (e.g., using Cavity Cleanser, Bisco Dental Products, Itasco, IL, USA). Some studies have shown success following disinfection of the pulpal exposure with 10% sodium hypochlorite followed by 10% hydrogen peroxide solutions (Matsuo et al. 1996). The exposure should be gently dried with a sterile cotton wool pledget. The calcium hydroxide is well adapted to the pulpal tissue and protected with a suitable covering layer of restorative material. It is essential that the restorative material prevent bacterial microleakage to ensure healing of the pulp. Fortunately, the pulp only becomes hyperemic when the carious lesion has extended to within a very short distance (0.25–0.3 mm) of the odontoblast layer (Shovelton 1968). However, where caries has penetrated into the pulp, considerable inflammation is present and direct pulp capping has a poor long-term success rate. Baume and Holz (1981) do not recommend direct pulp capping of carious pulpal exposures. If the pulp eventually becomes necrotic, the interim deposition of reactionary dentin and any infection can worsen the expected outcome from endodontic procedures.

Recently, step-wise excavation of caries in two stages has been recommended in those large carious lesions with reversible pulpitis. The technique involves careful removal of all peripheral caries in the cavity, leaving soft, wet, and infected dentin on the dentinal pulpal surface. The pale-colored pulpal dentin is covered with calcium hydroxide and a glass ionomer restoration and left for 6–12 months. After this time, the cavity is reentered and the pulpal dentinal surface will have become darker and harder. The technique has a reduced risk of pulpal exposure.

2.3.7
The Use of Calcium Hydroxide in Direct Pulp Capping

Opponents of the use of calcium hydroxide claim that the pulp-capping material has a tendency to dissolve, has the disadvantage of no adhesion to dentin, composite, or dentin bonding agents, and forms dentin bridges that are porous (Cox et al. 1996). They claim that calcium hydroxide has poor long-term therapeutic potential. However, studies by Matsuo et al. (1996) showed that when used as a direct pulp-capping material, calcium hydroxide has a success rate of about 80% when the patients were followed up for over 18 months. This was despite the inclusion of patients with lingering pain to a thermal stimulus at the start of the study. This study found that a poor success rate (56%) resulted from extensive bleeding at the pulpal exposure, which is an indication of pulpal inflammation. Blood between the calcium hydroxide pulp cap and the dentin surface probably accentuates inflammation. Long-term failure of calcium hydroxide pulp-capping procedures is associated with microleakage and penetration of bacteria through the porous dentin bridge into the pulp. Calcium hydroxide may have an important effect in stimulating tertiary dentin by releasing growth factors locked in the dentin matrix. The released growth factors, such as transforming growth factor-β, stimulate pulpal cells to differentiate directly into odontoblast-like cells and their precursors and lay down tertiary dentin. Rutherford et al. (1992) have shown that adding growth factor combinations (mixtures of recombinant human platelet-derived growth factor and insulin-like growth factor), can induce a favorable in vivo bone-healing response. When the same combination of growth factors was added to calcium hydroxide, improved healing of apical perforations was found in dogs (Kim et al. 2001). Exogenously applied enamel matrix molecules have also been shown to induce rapid pulpal wound healing in pulpotomized teeth and have been shown to be more effective than calcium hydroxide (Nakamura et al. 2004). Enamel matrix proteins recruit new odontoblasts from pulpal stem cells, whereas calcium hydroxide causes the stimulation of reparative dentin by adjacent preexisting odontoblasts. Enamel matrix proteins also have antibacterial properties (Spahr et al. 2002), which will also aid healing. Bone sialoprotein also induces homogeneous and well-mineralized tertiary dentin (Goldberg et al. 2001). There is much research interest in developing bioactive molecules for dentin regeneration, but as yet these molecules are expensive and clinically untested.

Alternative hydrophilic materials such as mineral trioxide aggregate react with sterile saline to form a highly biocompatible material when placed on pulpal tissue. Whether this material eventually displaces calcium hydroxide seems unlikely as the material has a prolonged setting reaction (about 4 hours) and has poor handling characteristics.

Calcium hydroxide has antibacterial properties, unlike some other proposed direct capping agents such as adhesive resins. In pulpal exposures contaminated with saliva, there is a greater likelihood of maintaining pulp vitality with calcium hydroxide than with adhesive resins. Light-activated forms of calcium hydroxide have less solubility, and further protection against dissolution can be afforded by placing a lining of glass ionomer and a sealed restoration over the calcium hydroxide. When adhesive resin is placed over the exposed pulp, the pulpal cells are in contact with diffusible monomers, which can have a direct toxic effect, but the in vivo concentration of these monomers in the pulp is not known.

2.3.8
The Foundation Restoration

Foundation (or build-up) restorations are not retained by undercut on the tooth. They are independently retained, because further removal of tooth substance may be necessary for crown preparation. Where coronal tooth destruction is severe, opposing walls may be absent and other forms of retention are necessary, such as pins, boxes, slots, and grooves.

Slots are prepared using an inverted cone bur (with head diameter 0.6 mm) and are placed 0.5 mm from the enamel-dentin junction. Grooves are placed using a 169L bur at the axiolingual and axiofacial line angles, 0.2 mm from the enamel-dentin junction. Boxes are used for additional retention by providing opposing vertical walls. The minimal gingival floor width of a box is 1.5 mm, but the necessary tooth preparation that this involves may make it an inadvisable form of retention, especially where the box must be extended too far subgingivally.

Self-threading pins (Fig. 2.22a) should be placed near the line angles of teeth, about 0.5–1 mm from the enamel-dentin junction. Because pins tend to weaken the overlying amalgam, it is better to avoid placing them below occlusal contacts to avoid the risk of amalgam fracture. The pinhole is prepared using a matched bur held parallel to the external surface of the tooth (Fig. 2.22b). The handpiece is also held in the long axis of the tooth, being careful to note any rotations or tooth misalignment. Pins weaken the dentin, and the stress concentration can cause fracture of the tooth. Therefore the minimum number of pins should be used (usually one per replacement cusp) with a minimum distance of 3–5 mm between pins. Several in vitro studies have found excellent fracture resistance and bond strengths of complex amalgams when pins were combined with dentin adhesives (Burgess et al. 1997; Sen et al. 2002). However, clinical trials would be needed to determine whether the favorable in vitro results were applicable in vivo.

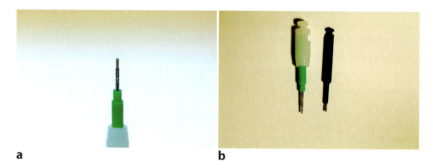

Fig. 2.22 (a) Self-threading pins should be placed in dentin in a direction parallel to the external surface of the tooth and about 0.5–1 mm from the enamel-dentin junction. (b) Self-threading pins are used with matching drills

2.3.9
Practical Aspects of Amalgam Retention

Pins are used where there are few opposing vertical cavity walls. However, they require about 3 mm of occlusogingival cavity height (Fig. 2.23), tend to cause microfractures in the dentin, and if used carelessly can traumatize the pulp or periodontal ligament. Where sufficient coronal substance is present, auxiliary forms of amalgam retention can be used, including boxes and slots.

2.3 Restorative Procedures

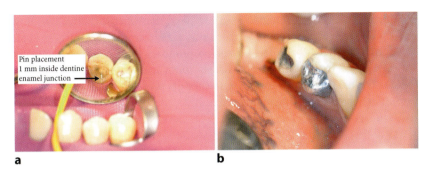

Fig. 2.23 (a) The minimum number of pins should be used (usually one per replacement cusp) with a minimum distance of 3–5 mm between pins. (b) The finished pin-retained amalgam. A 1-mm width of amalgam must cover the pin for the restoration to have good strength

Essentially, these forms of retention rely on near-parallel or undercut cavity walls. Creating additional opposing parallel walls will improve retention (e.g., in the compound class I amalgam) by utilizing the buccal and lingual grooves of molar teeth.

Amalgapins are 1.5- to 2-mm-deep channels prepared in dentin with a pear-shaped bur (No. 330 bur) and then filled with amalgam. The channels have a maximum diameter of 1 mm and the orifice is beveled to prevent the build up of damaging stress during oral function. With amalgapins the resistance to occlusal forces is comparable to pins once the amalgam has set, but immediately after insertion of the amalgam its retention and resistance are weak.

Circumferential grooving is an extension of the amalgapin preparation that involves placing a groove with a No. $33\frac{1}{2}$ inverted cone bur in dentin, about 0.5–1 mm from the amelodentinal junction. The depth of the groove is 0.75 mm, the full length of the bur head.

2.3.10
Pins vs Bonded Restorations

Summitt et al. (2001) found no difference in the clinical performance after 5 years of 60 complex amalgam restorations (each replacing at least one cusp) retained with either self-threading pins or a 4-methacryloxyethyl trimellitate anhydride (4-META) resin. Those in favor of bonded amalgams maintain that they allow smaller cavity preparations, avoid the use of pins, and reduce the incidence of secondary caries by preventing marginal microleakage. Most in vitro studies have found that bonded amalgams have a resistance to failure that is similar to that of pin-retained amalgam, and that when adhesive bonding was combined with pin retention there was an additive effect (Burgess et al. 1997; Imbery et al. 1995). The corrosion products from bonded amalgams may be less likely to infiltrate the adjacent tooth and cause gray staining, but there is little experimental evidence to support this. There are no long-term proven benefits to bonding amalgam.

2.3.11
Amalgam Bonding Procedure

The amalgam surface should be roughened. The adhesion of fresh amalgam to old does not match the cohesive strength of the original restoration, so auxiliary retention such as dovetails and boxes must be used. An adhesive 4-META resin can also be used to improve the bond strength (Amalgambond-Plus; Parkell, Farmingdale, NY, USA). The dentin activator is applied to the dentin for 30 s, rinsed, and dried, followed by application of the adhesive agent, which is air dried for 30 s. The base, catalyst, and high-performance additive powder is mixed and applied to the cavity, and amalgam is condensed immediately.

Where amalgam bonding resins are used, the minimal amount of liquid bonding resin should be used because it weakens the amalgam if used excessively. Excess resin will also be extruded by the condensed amalgam and bond to the matrix band, making the band difficult to remove without damaging the amalgam restoration. After placement of the bonding resin, the amalgam must be condensed immediately.

Smales and Wetherell (2000) found few advantages in survival of bonded amalgams over 5 years. Other authors have found poor bond strengths with using adhesive resin bonding to repair amalgam. The inherent esthetic disadvantages of bonded amalgam restorations severely limit the application of this technique, particularly when the results of bonded composite resin restorations are so favorable. Macpherson and Smith (1994) showed in an in vitro study that layered restorations with glass ionomer replacing dentin and composite resin replacing the enamel, performed as well as pin-retained amalgams. These layered restorations had mean fracture loads that were well within tolerance limits experienced intraorally (300 N).

Large amalgam restorations are an excellent, cost-effective method of treating patients. They are not the automatically inferior alternative to providing crowns. Kelly and Smales (2004) found in a survey of three private dental practices that "the full gold crown is 3.4 times, the posterior ceramometal crown is 3.6 times and the cast gold onlay is 4.6 times more expensive than the class II cusp-overlay amalgam".

2.3.12
The Use of Base Materials

The traditional use of base materials involved their extensive use as a dentin replacement, and as pulpal protection. The acidity of certain restorative materials was thought to be a considerable pulpal insult, but it is now accepted that bacterial penetration around restorations (microleakage) is responsible for much postoperative inflammation and sensitivity. Thermal conduction of cold and hot stimuli through amalgam to the pulpal nerves was also thought to necessitate a thick lining material under the amalgam to act as an insulator. This is incorrect as pulpal nerve stimulation results from fluid movement in the dentinal tubules, and postoperative thermal sensitivity can be much reduced by blocking the tubules with a desensitizing solution, dentin-bonding resins, or radiopaque resin modified glass ionomer (such as Vitrebond, manufactured by 3M ESPE, MN, USA). There is little rationale for using lining materials with a thickness greater than 0.5 mm, as the overlying amalgam, ceramic, or resin composite restorative material will lack sufficient bulk and will be weakened.

References

Atkinson DR, Cobb CM, Killoy WJ. The effect of an air-powder abrasive system on in vitro root surfaces. J Periodontol 1984; 55:13–18.

Banerjee A, Kidd EA, Watson TF. In vitro validation of carious dentin removed using different excavation criteria. Am J Dent 2003; 16:228–230.

Baume LJ, Holz J. Long term clinical assessment of direct pulp capping. Int Dent J 1981; 31:251–260.

Baysan A, Lynch E. Effect of ozone on the oral microbiota and clinical severity of primary root caries. Am J Dent 2004; 17:56–60.

Baysan A, Whiley RA, Lynch E. Antimicrobial effect of a novel ozone-generating device on micro-organisms associated with primary root carious lesions in vitro. Caries Res 2000; 34:498–501.

Bettner MD, Beiswanger MA, Miller CH, Palenik CJ. Effect of ultrasonic cleaning on microorganisms. Am J Dent 1998; 11:185–188.

Bonecker M, Toi C, Cleaton-Jones P. Mutans streptococci and lactobacilli in carious dentine before and after Atraumatic Restorative Treatment. J Dent 2003; 31:423–428.

Boston DW. New device for selective dentin caries removal. Quintessence Int 2003; 34:678–685.

Bulut G, Zekioglu O, Eronat C, Bulut H. Effect of Carisolv on the human dental pulp: a histological study. J Dent. 2004; 32:309–314.

Burgess JO, Alvarez A, Summitt JB. Fracture resistance of complex amalgam restorations. Oper Dent 1997; 22:128–132.

Burke FJT, Wilson NHF, Cheung SW, Mjor IA. Influence of patient factors on age of restorations at failure and reasons for their placement and replacement. J Dent 2001; 29:317–324.

Cipriano TM, Ferreira Santos JF. Clinical behavior of repaired amalgam restorations: a two-year study. J Prosthet Dent 1995; 73:8–11.

Cox CF, Subay RK, Ostro E, Suzuki S, Suzuki SH. Tunnel defects in dentin bridges: their formation following direct pulp capping. Oper Dent 1996; 21:4–11.

Cudd LA, Burrows GE, Clarke CR Pharmacokinetics and toxicity of tolonium chloride in sheep. Vet Hum Toxicol 1996; 38:329–332.

Dederich DN, Bushick RD; ADA Council on Scientific Affairs and Division of Science; Journal of the American Dental Association. Lasers in dentistry: separating science from hype. J Am Dent Assoc 2004; 135:204–212.

Dostalova T, Jelinkova H, Krejsa O, Hamal K, Kubelka J, Prochazka S, Himmlova L. Dentin and pulp response to Erbium:YAG laser ablation: a preliminary evaluation of human teeth. J Clin Laser Med Surg 1997; 15:117–121.

Eguro T, Maeda T, Otsuki M, Nishimura Y, Katsuumi I, Tanaka H. Adhesion of Er:YAG laser-irradiated dentin and composite resins: application of various treatments on irradiated surface. Lasers Surg Med 2002; 30:267–272.

Elderton RJ, Davis M. Restorative dental treatment in the General Dental Service in Scotland. Br Dent J 1984; 157:196–200.

Elderton RJ. The prevalence of failure of restorations: a literature review. J Dent 1976a; 4:207–210.

Elderton RJ. The causes of failure of restorations; a literature review. J Dent 1976b; 4:257–262.

Evans DJ, Matthews S, Pitts NB, Longbottom C, Nugent ZJ. A clinical evaluation of an Erbium:YAG laser for dental cavity preparation. Br Dent J 2000; 24; 188:677–679.

Foster LV. Three year in vivo investigation to determine the progression of approximal primary carious lesions extending into dentine. Br Dent J 1998; 185:353–357.

Frencken JE, Van't Hof MA, Van Amerongen WE, Holmgren CJ. Effectiveness of single-surface ART restorations in the permanent dentition: a meta-analysis. J Dent Res 2004; 83:120–123.

Fusayama T. Clinical guide for removing caries using a caries-detecting solution. Quintessence Int 1988; 19:397–401.

Gao W, Peng D, Smales RJ, Yip KH. Comparison of atraumatic restorative treatment and conventional restorative procedures in a hospital clinic: evaluation after 30 months. Quintessence Int 2003; 34:31–37.

Going RE, Loesche WJ, Grainger DA, Syed SA. The viability of microorganisms in carious lesions five years after covering with a fissure sealant. J Am Dent Assoc 1978; 97:455–462.

Goldberg J, Tanzer J, Munster E, Amara J, Thal F, Birkhed D. Cross-sectional clinical evaluation of recurrent caries, restoration of marginal integrity, and oral hygiene status. J Am Dent Assoc 1981; 102:635–641.

Goldberg M, Six N, Decup F, Buch D, Soheili Majd E, Lasfargues JJ, Salih E, Stanislawski L. Application of bioactive molecules in pulp-capping situations. Adv Dent Res 2001; 15:91–95.

Handelman SL, Washburn F, Wopperer P. Two-year report of sealant effect on bacteria in dental caries. J Am Dent Assoc 1976; 93:967–970.

Hasselrot L. Tunnel restorations in permanent teeth: a 7-year follow-up study. Swed Dent J 1998; 22; 1–7.

Hintze H, Wenzel A, Danielsen B. Behaviour of approximal carious lesions assessed by clinical examination after tooth separation and radiography: a 2.5 year longitudinal study in young adults. Caries Res 1999; 33:415–422.

Hoke JA, Burkes EJ Jr, Gomes ED, Wolbarsht ML. Erbium:YAG (2.94 mum) laser effects on dental tissues J Laser Appl 1990; 2:61–65.

Honkala S, Honkala E. Atraumatic dental treatment among Finnish elderly persons. J Oral Rehabil 2002; 29:435–440.

Imbery TA, Burgess JO, Batzer RC. Comparing the resistance of dentin bonding agents and pins in amalgam restorations. J Am Dent Assoc 1995; 126:753–759.

Jahn KR, Geitel B, Kostka E, Wischnewski R, Roulet JF. Tensile bond strength of composite to air-abraded enamel. Adhes Dent 1999; 1:25–30.

Jokstad A, Mjör IA. Analyses of long-term clinical behavior of class-II amalgam restorations. Acta Odont Scand 1991; 49:47–63.

Kakaboura A, Masouras C, Staikou O, Vougiouklakis G. A comparative clinical study on the Carisolv caries removal method. Quintessence Int 2003; 34:269–271.

Kavvadia K, Karagianni V, Polychronopoulou A, Papagiannouli L. Primary teeth caries removal using the Carisolv chemomechanical method: a clinical trial. Pediatr Dent 2004; 26:23–28.

Kelly PG, Smales RJ. Long-term cost-effectiveness of single indirect restorations in selected dental practices. Br Dent J 2004; 196:639–643.

Kidd EA, Joyston-Bechal S, Smith MM, Allan R, Howe L, Smith SR. The use of a caries detector dye in cavity preparation. Br Dent J 1989; 167:132–134.

Kidd EAM. How 'clean' must a cavity be before restoration? Caries Res 2004; 38:305–313.

Kim M, Kim B, Yoon S. Effect on the healing of periapical perforations in dogs of the addition of growth factors to calcium hydroxide. J Endod 2001; 27:734–737.

Klein H, Fuks A, Eidelman E, Chosak A. Partial pulpotomy following complicated crown fracture in permanent incisors: a clinical and radiographical study. J Pedod 1985; 9:142–147.

Kohns P, Zhou P, Stormann R. Effective laser ablation of enamel and dentine without thermal side effects. J Laser Appl 1997; 9:171–174.

Laurell KA, Carpenter W, Daugherty D, Beck M. Histopathologic effects of kinetic cavity preparation for the removal of enamel and dentin. An in vivo animal study. Oral Surg Oral Med Oral Pathol Oral Radiol Endod 1995; 80:214–225.

Macpherson LC, Smith BG. Replacement of missing cusps: an in vitro study. J Dent 1994; 22:118–120.

Malmstrom HS, Chaves Y, Moss ME. Patient preference: conventional rotary handpieces or air abrasion for cavity preparation. Oper Dent 2003; 28:667–671.

Mandari GJ, Frencken JE, van't Hof MA. Six-year success rates of occlusal amalgam and glass-ionomer restorations placed using three minimal intervention approaches. Caries Res 2003; 37:246–253.

Matsuo T, Nakanishi T, Shimizu H, Ebisu S. A clinical study of direct pulp capping applied to carious-exposed pulps. J Endod 1996; 22:551–556.

McDaniel RJ, Davis RD, Murchison DF, Cohen RB. Causes of failure among cuspal-coverage amalgam restorations: a clinical survey. J Am Dent Assoc 2000; 131:173–177.

Merret CW, Elderton RJ. An in vitro study of restorative treatment decisions and dental caries. Br Dent J 1984; 157:128–133.

Mestrener SR, Holland R, Dezan E Jr. Influence of age on the behavior of dental pulp of dog teeth after capping with an adhesive system or calcium hydroxide. Dent Traumatol 2003; 19:255–261.

Mount GJ, Ngo H. Minimal intervention: early lesions. Quintessence Int. 2000; 31:535–546.

Nakamura Y, Slaby I, Matsumoto K, Ritchie HH, Lyngstadaas SP. Immunohistochemical characterization of rapid dentin formation induced by enamel matrix derivative. Calcif Tissue Int 2004; 75:243–252.

Nuckles DB, Draughn RA, Smith TI. Evaluation of an adhesive system for amalgam repair: bond strength and porosity. Quintessence Int 1994; 25:829–833.

Otsuki M, Eguro T, Maeda T, Tanaka H. Comparison of the bond strength of composite resin to Er:YAG laser irradiated human enamel pre-treated with various methods in vitro. Lasers Surg Med 2002; 30:351–359.

Palma-Dibb RG, de Castro CG, Ramos RP, Chimello DT, Chinelatti MA. Bond strength of glass-ionomer cements to caries-affected dentin. J Adhes Dent 2003; 5:57–62.

Paterson FM, Paterson RC, Watts A, Blinkhorn AS. Initial stages in the development of valid criteria for the replacement of amalgam restorations. J Dent 1995; 23:137–143.

Petersilka GJ, Bell M, Häberlein I, Mehl A, Hickel R, Flemmig TF: In vitro evaluation of novel low abrasive air polishing powders. J Clin Periodontol 2003; 30:9–13.

Pitts NB, Rimmer PA. An in vivo comparison of radiographic and directly assessed clinical caries status of posterior approximal surfaces in primary and permanent teeth. Caries Res 1992; 26:146–152.

Rafique S, Fiske J, Banerjee A. Clinical trial of an air-abrasion/chemomechanical operative procedure for the restorative treatment of dental patients. Caries Res 2003; 37:360–364.

Rickard G, Richardson R, Johnson T, McColl D, Hooper L. Ozone therapy for the treatment of dental caries. Cochrane Database Syst Rev 2004; 3:CD004153.

Ricketts D. Management of the deep carious lesion and the vital pulp dentine complex. Br Dent J 2001; 191:606–610.

Rutherford RB, Niekrash CE, Kennedy JE, Charette MF. Platelet-derived and insulin-like growth factors stimulate regeneration of periodontal attachment in monkeys. J Periodontal Res 1992; 27:285–290.

Sen D, Nayir E, Çetiner F. Shear bond strength of amalgam reinforced with a bonding agent and/or dentin pins. J Prosthet Dent 2002; 87:446–450.

Shovelton DS. A study of deep carious dentin. Int Dent J 1968; 18:392–405.

Smales RJ, Hawthorne WS. Long-term survival of repaired amalgams, recemented crowns and gold castings. Oper Dent 2004; 29:249–253.

Smales RJ, Wetherell JD. Review of bonded amalgam restorations, and assessment in a general practice over five years. Oper Dent 2000; 25:374–381.

References

Smales RJ, Yip HK. The atraumatic restorative treatment (ART) approach for the management of dental caries. Quintessence Int 2002; 33:427–432.

Spahr A, Lyngstadaas SP, Boeckh C, Andersson C, Podbielski A, Haller B. Effect of the enamel matrix derivative Emdogain on the growth of periodontal pathogens in vitro. J Clin Periodontol 2002; 29:62–72.

Summitt JB, Burgess JO, Berry TG, Robbins JW, Osborne JW, Haveman CW. The performance of bonded vs. pin-retained complex amalgam restorations: a five-year clinical evaluation. J Am Dent Assoc 2001; 132:923–931.

Thomas CC, Land MF, Albin-Wilson SM, Stewart GP. Caries detection accuracy by multiple clinicians and techniques Gen Dent 2000; 48:334–338.

van Nieuwenhuysen JP, D'Hoore W, Carvalho J, Qvist V. Long-term evaluation of extensive restorations in permanent teeth. J Dent 2003; 31:395–405.

Whitworth CL, Martin MV, Gallagher M, Worthington HV. A comparison of decontamination methods used for dental burs. Br Dent J 2004; 197:635–640.

Williams JA, Pearson GJ, Colles MJ, Wilson M. The effect of variable energy input from a novel light source on the photoactivated bactericidal action of toluidine blue O on Streptococcus mutans. Caries Res 2003; 37:190–193.

Yazici AR, Atilla P, Ozgunaltay G, Muftuoglu S. In vitro comparison of the efficacy of Carisolv and conventional rotary instrument in caries removal. J Oral Rehabil 2003 30:1177–1182.

Yip HK, Stevenson AG, Beeley JA. The specificity of caries detector dyes in cavity preparation. Br Dent J 1994; 176:417–421.

Young C, Bongenhielm U. A randomised, controlled and blinded histological and immunohistochemical investigation of Carisolv on pulp tissue. J Dent 2001; 29:275–281.

3 Posterior Resin Composite Restorations

Small pits and fissures with minimal caries can be treated very conservatively and restored directly with good esthetics using composite resin. In addition, the remaining fissures can be protected with a resin sealant. The main contraindication to restoring the tooth with composite resin is an inability to isolate the tooth from salivary contamination, which would prevent the composite forming an effective bond to the tooth structure. The wear resistance of posterior composites has improved so that these materials have wear that is comparable to that of amalgam (Mair 1995). Wear is of little concern with these minimal restorations, as occlusal forces are also directed to the adjacent enamel. The modern small-particle composites have an improved abrasion resistance and can be polished easily.

The major advantage of adhesive resin composite restorations is their conservative nature. Amalgam preparations require removing sufficient tooth substance to obtain adequate retention to resist applied occlusal loads; even the most minimal occlusal amalgam preparations need to be extended by 0.5 mm into dentin with occlusally converging walls. When using composite resin with an acid-etch bonding technique it is not necessary to remove all unsupported enamel, except weak, friable tissue, as the bonded restoration strengthens the tooth. Caries in dentin spreads laterally along the enamel-dentin junction, often producing an undermined enamel layer of normal thickness (Fig. 3.1). With amalgam it can be difficult to prevent voids forming in these less accessible areas, whereas composite restorations can be easily packed into these areas and bonded.

A major disadvantage of composite resin is the polymerization shrinkage these materials undergo following light curing. The extent of polymerization shrinkage is greater with microfilled resins, but due to plastic flow relaxation some of the polymerization shrinkage stress is dissipated and not transferred to the adhesive bond. The likelihood of gap formation and failure of the adhesive bond is dependent upon the "C" or configuration-factor (i.e., the ratio of bonded to unbonded surface in a restoration). An increase in the C factor results in a greater contraction stress because the possibility of plastic

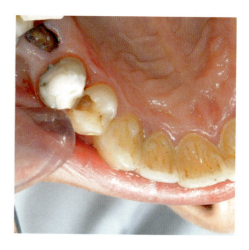

Fig. 3.1 When restoring interproximal carious lesions with adhesively retained composite resin restorations, it is not necessary to remove all unsupported enamel. Occlusal extension to form a lock or keyway is also unnecessary

flow of the composite resin is reduced. Large contraction stresses are then applied directly to the adhesive bond. The most unfavorable situation is found where there is a large bonded surface:free unbonded surface ratio, such as with class I and II cavities.

3.1
Ramped Curing Lights

Ramped light-curing units use a low light intensity ($< 400\,mW/cm^2$) during the initial phase of composite resin polymerization so that plastic flow can occur. This tends to reduce the stress on the adhesive bond. Argon lasers (emitting blue light at 488 nm) are able to initiate polymerization of the resin composite, but the reduced duration of cure and the increased depth of polymerization do not compensate for the increased stress on the adhesive bond.

3.2
Ceramic Inserts

Ceramic inserts reduce the amount of polymerization shrinkage by reducing the bulk of resin composite needed to restore the tooth. The inserts can be very useful when used with resin composite to replace a large, failed amalgam restoration. Figure 3.2 shows one commercially available ceramic inlay system (Cerana). Using a size-matched diamond bur (Fig. 3.3a), the cavity is prepared in the usual way (Fig. 3.3b). The cavity is etched and bond resin applied. Resin

3.2 Ceramic Inserts

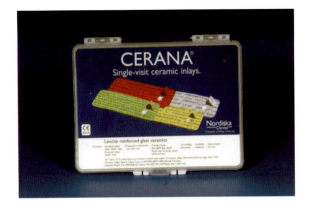

Fig. 3.2 This commercially available ceramic inlay system reduces the amount of resin composite required, and therefore its shrinkage due to polymerization

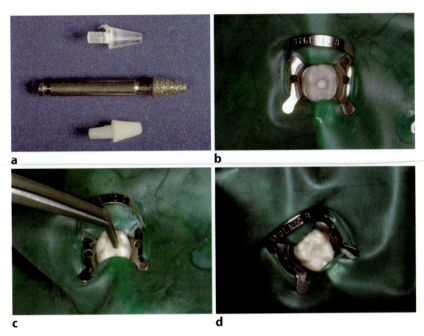

Fig. 3.3 (a) The cavity is prepared using a size-matched bur and etched. Primer/bond and resin composite are applied and cured. The clear curing cone is used in large cavities to assist with light-curing of the deepest areas of resin composite. The white ceramic insert is matched for the size of the bur. (b) The ceramic insert technique is best used where the cavity is large and requires a considerable amount of resin composite, or where the cavity has a large "C" factor. (c) Bonding resin is applied to the ceramic inlay and is pressed into the cavity. Excess resin composite is removed and the restoration is light-cured for 40 s. (d) The occlusal contour of the ceramic/resin composite restoration is adjusted

composite is applied to the cavity, filling it to the enamel-dentin junction. The clear curing cone can be inserted into large cavities with severe undercut to assist with light-curing the resin composite. Bonding resin is applied to the white, pre-etched, presilanized Cerana inlay and pressed into the cavity (Fig. 3.3c). Excess resin composite is removed and the restoration is light-cured for 40 s. The occlusal contour of the inlay is shaped to be harmonious with the surrounding enamel and the occlusion adjusted (Fig. 3.3d). Following removal of the excess material, the restoration is cured for a further 40 s. The restoration is finally polished. Ceramic inserts bonded with resin composite show no adverse microleakage effects (Kuramoto et al. 2000).

3.3
Nanotechnology

Higher filler loading has been used in the past to reduce polymerization shrinkage, but the large particles used inevitably resulted in poor polishability. Microfill resins that contain silica nanoparticles are weaker, often insufficiently radiopaque, and perform poorly in the posterior region of the mouth. New developments in resin composites have reduced polymerization volumetric shrinkage to less than 2% by incorporating high filler loading with particles of different sizes. With these new "nanocomposites," the esthetics are better as the resin composite blends with the surrounding tooth enamel, while strength is not compromised.

The new nanocluster resin composites have less polymerization shrinkage and better physical properties. They also produce a better polish because a nanosized particle is larger than the wavelength of light and is not reflected by the particle, so therefore appears more translucent.

3.4
"Total Etch" Technique

The "total etch" technique describes the simultaneous etching of both enamel and dentin. The technique does not harm the tooth, as very little, if any, acid penetrates the dentin and pulp, unless there is very little remaining dentin (Hebling et al. 1999). The principal of dentin bonding is that the smear layer is removed with decalcification of the intertubular and peritubular dentin. Inevitably, there is an increase in the permeability of the dentin and a larger outflow of pulpal fluid from the dentinal tubules. The hypertonicity of the acid gel causes the further increased outflow of pulpal fluid, which tends to dilute the acid. The dissolved hydroxyapatite also tends to buffer the conditioner so that increasing the duration of conditioner application does not cause a proportional increase in the depth of dentin demineralization. Application of the conditioner removes intertubular mineral to a depth of about 5 μm, widens the tubules, and causes the formation of a demineralized collagen meshwork, which is susceptible to collapse if dried excessively. Dentin bonding agents contain a primer (such as hydroxyethyl methacrylate, HEMA, or 4-META) and an adhesive monomer resin. The function of the primer is to penetrate into the collagen framework and copolymerize with the resin. This resin-infiltrated layer is called the hybrid layer. The entanglement of the resins in the microporous dentin provides much of the retention for the composite resin. A thick (125 μm) layer of adhesive resin may have advantages over a thinner layer because it will stretch during polymerization of the composite resin, tending to relieve polymerization stress at the margin.

Over-etching the dentin results in the resin being unable to penetrate to the full depth of the demineralization. This leaves a zone beneath the hybrid layer that may be susceptible to nanoleakage (Paul et al. 1999). In addition, there is a reduction in bond strength of the subsequently applied resin composite.

3.5
Fissure Sealants

Fissure sealants are indicated to protect the occlusal surface of newly erupted teeth in caries-prone children. Isolation of these teeth with a rubber dam may be difficult, and cotton wool rolls may be used instead. Fissure sealants are an effective form of treatment at preventing caries, despite the poor retention rates in some studies. Gibson et al. (1982), using a split half-mouth design, showed that fissure sealants caused a 51% reduction in caries, despite about only two-thirds remaining intact. Presumably, resin tags remained in the depth of the fissure, but were invisible to the examining dentist. The age of the patient influences the ease at which isolation of the tooth can be obtained, which in turn will influence the retention of the fissure sealant. Even in young children, some studies have shown excellent retention rates. In 7 year-old children, the retention of a glass ionomer fissure sealant in the deciduous molars varied from 50 to 75% after 1 year (Poulsen et al. 2003). However, placing fissure sealants successfully is highly dependent upon operator skill (Holst et al. 1998).

The effect of inadvertently sealing dentinal caries is to reduce the number of viable bacteria in the lesion so that further tooth destruction does not occur. Going et al. (1978) and Handelman et al. (1976) found that applying a fissure sealant to active caries would render the lesion inactive in the vast majority of cases, provided the restoration remained sealed.

Technique for Fissure Sealant Placement

The tooth is isolated using a rubber dam and the fissures cleaned with a slurry of pumice applied with a bristle brush in a slow-speed handpiece. The enamel is etched with phosphoric acid solution, rinsed, and dried. The sealant is then applied, worked into the fissures with a brush, and light-cured for 20 s. On removing the rubber dam, the occlusion is checked with articulating paper (Fig. 3.4).

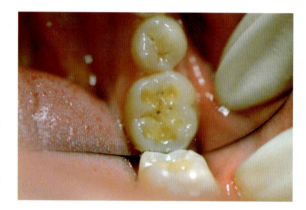

Fig. 3.4 Fissure sealants can be used in combination with localized excavation of carious pits for preventive resin restoration

3.6
Preventive Resin Restorations

These restorations are indicated when occlusal caries has involved a minimal amount of dentin. The technique involves isolating the tooth using a rubber dam. The fissure is investigated using a no. 0.5 round diamond bur, to a depth of about 1 mm. When this initial phase of cavity preparation is complete, the extent of caries can be assessed more easily and a decision taken as to whether to extend the cavity to the enamel-dentin junction. Any caries is removed with a small, no. $\frac{1}{2}$ round bur. Overhanging enamel is left in situ as the adhesive resin composite will provide strength to the tooth. The enamel and dentin are etched, washed, and dried (but the dentin remains moist and glistening). The enamel/dentin bonding agent (primers and adhesives) is applied with a small applicator. The bonding agent is polymerized for about 10 s. Composite resin is then applied incrementally and light-cured. The remaining etched fissures and the composite resin can be sealed with a thin layer of fissure sealant. The rubber dam is removed and the occlusion checked with articulating paper and adjusted where necessary.

3.7
Minimal Class II Restorations

Following entry into the approximal region through the marginal ridge and removal of caries, extension of the cavity through the occlusal fissure may not be necessary. Retention can be provided by grooves in dentin at the pulpoaxial line angles. These grooves can be extended to the occlusal surface.

3.8
Posterior Composite Resin Restoration

Following the application of local anesthesia, the tooth is isolated with a rubber dam. The larger class I tooth preparation has an initial depth of about 1.5 mm, just penetrating into the dentin. The caries is removed from the enamel-dentin junction. Small class I cavities will have sufficient retention and resistance form from the adhesive restoration so that occlusally converging walls and flat pulpal floors may not be necessary, but where the restoration becomes more extensive then these features should be incorporated. Beveled occlusal margins are contraindicated because the thin margin of composite resin is easily lost during function, leaving a margin that quickly becomes stained. However, buccal and lingual grooves, where the occlusal contacts are lighter, can be given a 0.5-mm-wide bevel.

The polymerization shrinkage of composite resin causes gap formation and postoperative sensitivity. Polymerization shrinkage with direct composite resin increases with the size of the cavity restoration, and together with the difficulties of restoring the proximal contact, increases the failure rate of restored large posterior cavities. With composite or ceramic inlays or onlays, only the resin cement lute undergoes polymerization shrinkage, thus resulting in good adaptation. In a study in which no dentin bonding system was used or any pretreatment of the inlay restoration after postcuring, 17.7% of direct inlays of direct composite restorations were unacceptable after 11 years (van Dijken 2000). By comparison, 27.3% of direct composite restorations were unacceptable after the same time. Durable bonding of resin composite to dentin is difficult to achieve, as some studies have shown incomplete penetration of the resin monomer into etched dentin, resulting in poor hybrid layer formation. Nanoleakage and water penetration may be a problem with some of the one-step, self-etching adhesive systems (Frankenberger et al. 2005), giving rise to hydrolytic degradation within the hybrid layer and a loss of adhesive bond strength of the resin composite with dentin (Okuda et al. 2002).

3.9
Direct Composite Resin Restorations

Once the caries has been removed, the remaining areas of the occlusal surface can be treated conservatively or with fissure sealants. Where necessary, calcium hydroxide can be used to protect the deepest areas of the cavity preparation, but this material has no adhesive properties. The enamel is etched for about 15 s, the dentin is etched for 10 s, and the etchant is washed off. The enamel surface is dried and the dentin moistened with a damp cotton wool pad. Overdrying etched dentin causes collapse of the exposed collagen fibers. The primer is applied and dried gently. The dentin surface should appear shiny. The adhesive bonding agent is applied and light-cured before applying the composite resin. The polymer chains of the polymerized resin wrap around the collagen fibers, providing the basis for the retention of the restoration. Lining materials such as flowable composite liners or resin-modified glass ionomers can provide a stress-absorbing layer immediately beneath the composite resin so that the effects of polymerization shrinkage, such as microleakage, are reduced.

GC-Fuji Lining LC Paste Pak (GC America, Alsip IL, USA) is a suitable two-paste, resin-modified glass ionomer for lining resin composite restorations. The material is dispensed from a cartridge using a special dispenser, mixed for 10 s and applied to the moist dentin tooth surface. It is then light-cured for 20 s. GC-Fuji Lining LC Paste bonds to dentin and resin composite, and absorbs the stresses caused by the polymerization shrinkage of resin composite materials.

For minimal cavities where polymerization shrinkage may not be great, intermediate stress-relieving materials between the resin composite and the tooth may not be necessary. In those circumstances, a satisfactory bond between the resin composite and the tooth may be provided by a dentin adhesive. There are many examples of these materials, but Clearfil SE Bond (J & S Davis and Kuraray Dental, Düsseldorf, Germany) is an example of a self-etching primer that simultaneously etches and primes dentin, and prepares enamel (Fig. 3.5). There is therefore no phosphoric acid etch stage, so washing and drying of the tooth is eliminated. The primer is applied, left for 20 s and dried with a gentle air flow. The bonding resin of Clearfil SE Bond is then applied, dried gently, and then light-cured for 10 s. The cavity is then ready to be restored with composite resin. The primer does not sufficiently condition uncut enamel, so if the resin is likely to cover the adjacent, unprepared tooth, then this surface should be first etched with phosphoric acid. Overfilling of the resin onto unetched enamel could cause marginal discoloration.

A high-filler-content composite resin is added in 2-mm-thick increments and cured. Composite resin restorations are contoured with 12-bladed finish-

3.9 Direct Composite Resin Restorations

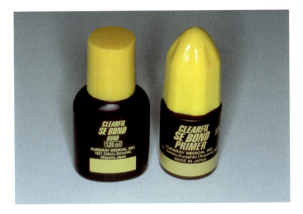

Fig. 3.5 This self-etching primer simultaneously etches and primes dentin. If the restoration involves enamel, then the enamel requires separate etching with phosphoric acid

ing burs and polished with rubber cups. Metallic instruments are unsuitable for placement of composites, as they easily stain the surface. Figure 3.6a illustrates the range of shapes of some disposable tips (Optra Sculpt from Ivoclar Vivadent) that can be used to carve posterior composite resin. They are detachable from the metal handle, which can be sterilized again for reuse (Fig. 3.6b). The rubber dam is removed and the occlusion checked with articulating paper. Any occlusal interferences are removed.

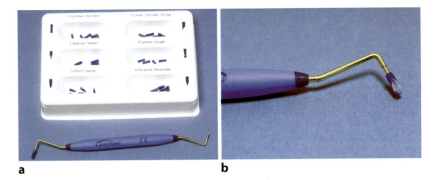

a b

Fig. 3.6 (a) Some disposable tips that can be used to carve posterior composite resin prior to curing (Optra Sculpt from Ivoclar Vivadent). (b) After carving of the resin composite is complete, the disposable tips are removed. The metal handle is sterilized for reuse

3.10
Studies of Direct Resin-Composite Restoration Survival

Van Nieuwenhuysen et al. (2003) found that composite resin was an unsuitable material with which to restore extensive cavity preparations in molar and premolar teeth. All retreatment was classed as failure, which resulted in a Kaplan-Meier median survival time of 7.8 years for resin restorations. This is in comparison to extensive amalgam restorations, which have been shown to be much more successful. However, extensive composite resin or amalgam restorations are cost-effective and can be easily repaired. The decision to repair an existing restoration rather than replace it should follow only after careful discussion of the treatment options with the patient. But the extent of active dentinal caries under a large restoration and the size of the new restoration can be difficult to predict.

El-Mowafy et al. (1994) analyzed the results of 16 studies in a meta-analysis involving eight different posterior composite materials, and found a generally high clinical performance. Other studies have demonstrated disappointing survival rates with multisurface composite resin restorations, but this may be related to the use of older technology resin composite systems. For example, Bentley and Drake (1986) found a survival rate of 40% in posterior composite restorations over 10 years. Collins et al. (1998) found that 8 years after placement, composite restorations in posterior teeth had failed at a rate two to three times greater than that of amalgam restorations.

3.11
Reasons for Failure of Extensive Direct Composite Resin Restorations

Where extensive posterior restorations are concerned, the adhesive bonding of composite resin restorations to tooth substance does not seem to provide much additional benefit. Bonded composite or porcelain inlays do not strengthen maxillary premolars previously weakened by large mesio-occlusal-distal (MOD) restorations. In a study by Friedl et al. (1995), fracture was the main reason for failure of four-surface composite resin restorations. With an extensive, directly applied composite resin restoration, it is difficult to perfect the occlusal contact in centric occlusion and lateral and protrusive jaw movements, and providing a tight interproximal contact can also be demanding (Fig. 3.7). This can result in premature contacts that can produce fracture of the tooth or restoration. Bayne et al. (1989) found that after 5 years, 30% of failures of posterior composites in their study were due to fracture. MOD restorations in maxillary premolars are weakest where the pulpal depth is increased, and in such cavities the tensile stresses at the bonded interface will be large, threatening debonding of the composite restorations (Lin et al. 2001).

With extensive direct composite restorations, contact of weak remaining cusps during working side contacts should be avoided to prevent tooth fracture (Fig. 3.8). Mesio-occlusodistal restorations in first molar teeth are particularly prone to further fracture (Patel and Burke 1995).

Some advocate that weakened premolar teeth should be restored by indirect onlay restorations, which will prevent cuspal deflection. The design of inlay and onlay restorations is independent of whether porcelain or composite resin is used. Inlay and onlay preparations require rounded internal line angles, and onlays a 1.5- to 2-mm reduction in cuspal height sufficient for the restorative material. Creating a path of insertion without undercut will result in more removal of tooth substance than with direct composite restorations.

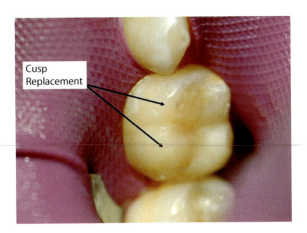

Fig. 3.7 With an extensive, directly applied resin-composite restoration, the restoration is easily left in premature occlusal contact. Providing a tight interproximal contact can also be demanding and placement of a matrix ban is therefore essential

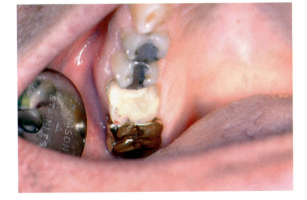

Fig. 3.8 With extensive direct composite restorations, contact of weak remaining cusps during working side contacts should be avoided to prevent tooth fracture. If the isolated distobuccal cusp of the first molar is left, further tooth fracture is likely

In smaller posterior restorations, discoloration of the margin and secondary caries are significant causes of failure, perhaps due to poor adaptation and gap formation at insertion and polymerization of the composite resin. But the success rate of these smaller restorations rival those of amalgam, especially where the composite resins have been placed under ideal conditions in university settings (Wilson et al. 1991). The success of posterior composite restorations is maximized where the external surface is surrounded by enamel and direct occlusal forces are avoided (Ferracane, 1992).

3.12
The "Sandwich" Technique

In the open-sandwich technique, glass ionomer restorative material forms the interproximal box of class II cavities and is extended occlusally from the gingival margin to just short of the contact point. Composite resin has better mechanical properties than glass ionomer and forms a protective covering layer. The technique is indicated in those patients with a high caries rate who require large posterior tooth restorations. The fluoride release by the glass ionomer is intended to prevent secondary caries by remineralizing the surrounding tooth. In addition, by reducing the bulk of composite resin that must be used, the polymerization shrinkage is also reduced.

The technique has been modified to replace the glass ionomer with resin modified glass ionomers (such as Vitremer Core Buildup/Restorative System, 3M Dental Products, St. Paul, MN, USA), which also release fluoride but have superior mechanical properties to traditional glass ionomer. Vitremer Core Buildup has a dual curing mechanism, with an extraoral working time of about 2.5 min. The material is also radiopaque, and so recurrent caries can be detected easily. Some studies have shown a reasonable success rate of these restorations in high-caries risk individuals (Andersson-Wenckert et al. 2004), although slow dissolution of the resin-modified glass ionomer, tooth and material fracture, and secondary caries were responsible for 19% of failed restorations after 6 years.

3.13
Packable Composite Resin Materials

Several manufacturers have introduced "packable" composite resin materials, which, it is claimed, make it easier during insertion to obtain a contact point with the adjacent teeth. These materials have a high viscosity, good wear resistance, and can be polished immediately after insertion. High filler

3.13 Packable Composite Resin Materials

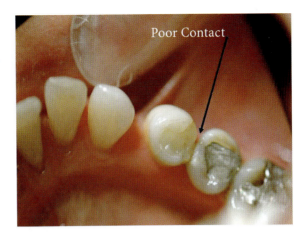

Fig. 3.9 An example of a poorly contoured resin-composite restoration. This can be prevented by contouring the metal matrix band with a burnisher, which improves the contact with the adjacent tooth

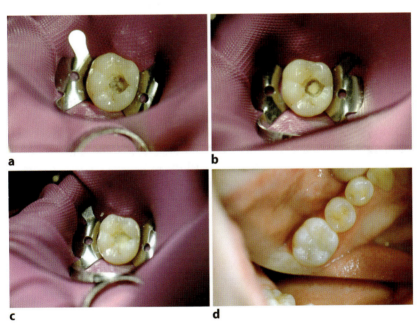

Fig. 3.10 (a) The caries is removed with minimal extension into the adjacent fissures. The pulpal floor is rounded. (b) A calcium hydroxide base was applied to the pulpal floor of the restoration, where it approached the pulp. (c) Calcium hydroxide is a weak, soluble material, therefore glass ionomer (or resin modified glass ionomer) base is placed over it. (d) The cavity was restored, polished, and the occlusion perfected

content composite resins have the least polymerization shrinkage, but even the packable composites shrink by 2–3% following light curing. These high filler content materials also have a decreased depth of cure, and bulk curing of these materials is not recommended. Some recommend placing a flowable composite in the box of a class II restoration to reach even the more inaccessible areas, followed by several increments of packable composite resin. Most flowable composites have adequate radiopacity for this indication, but the distance of the material on the gingival floor of the cavity from the curing light may require that an extended curing time of at least 40 s duration be used.

Conventional resin composites often lack sufficient viscosity to form a good contact point in extensive posterior restorations (Fig. 3.9). However, the adhesive bond of resin composite to the enamel provides fracture resistance to the molar cusps. Following caries removal (Fig. 3.10a), it is only necesary to remove any friable enamel prior to restoration (Fig. 3.10b,c). This results in a conservative restoration (Fig. 3.10d).

3.14
New Developments in Resin-Composite Technology

Future progress in composite technology will involve development of "shrink-free" composite resins. Silorane composites have low shrinkage ($< 1\%$) and good biocompatibility, and their mechanical properties are comparable to those of conventional methacrylate-based resins (Guggenberger and Weinmann 2000). The low shrinkage following polymerization ensures excellent marginal adaptation.

References

Andersson-Wenckert IE, van Dijken JW, Kieri C. Durability of extensive Class II open-sandwich restorations with a resin-modified glass ionomer cement after 6 years. Am J Dent 2004; 17:43–50.

Bayne SC, Taylor DF, Robertson TM et al. Long-term clinical failures in posterior composites. J Dent Res 1989; 68:185, Abst 32.

Bentley C, Drake CW. Longevity of restorations in a dental school clinic. J Dent Educ 1986; 50:594–600.

Collins CJ, Bryant RW, Hodge KL. A clinical evaluation of posterior composite resin restorations: 8-year findings. J Dent 1998; 26:311–317.

El-Mowafy OM, Lewis DW, Benmergui C, Levinton C. Meta-analysis on long-term clinical performance of posterior composite restorations. J Dent 1994; 22:33–43.

Ferracane JL. Using posterior composites appropriately. J Am Dent Assoc 1992; 123: 53–58.

References

Frankenberger R, Pashley DH, Reich SM, Lohbauer U, Petschelt A, Tay FR. Characterisation of resin-dentine interfaces by compressive cyclic loading. Biomaterials 2005; 26:2043–2052.

Gibson GB, Richardson AS, Waldman R. The effectiveness of a chemically polymerized sealant in preventing occlusal caries: five-year results. Pediatr Dent 1982; 4:309–310.

Going RE, Loesche WJ, Grainger DA, Syed SA. The viability of microorganisms in carious lesions five years after covering with a fissure sealant. J Am Dent Assoc 1978; 97:455–462.

Guggenberger R, Weinmann W. Exploring beyond methacrylates. Am J Dent 2000; 13:82D–84D.

Handelman SL, Washburn F, Wopperer P. Two-year report of sealant effect on bacteria in dental caries. J Am Dent Assoc 1976; 93:967–970.

Hebling J, Giro EM, Costa CA. Human pulp response after an adhesive system application in deep cavities. J Dent 1999; 27:557–564.

Holst A, Braune K, Sullivan A. A five-year evaluation of fissure sealants applied by dental assistants. Swed Dent J 1998; 22:195–201.

Kuramoto M Jr, Matos AB, Matson E, Eduardo CP, Powers JM. Microleakage of resin-based composite restorations with ceramic inserts. Am J Dent 2000; 13:311–314.

Lin CL, Chang CH, Ko CC. Multifactorial analysis of an MOD restored human premolar using auto-mesh finite element approach. J Oral Rehabil 2001; 28:576–585.

Mair LH. Wear patterns in two amalgams and three posterior composites after 5 years clinical service. J Dent 1995; 23:107–112.

Okuda M, Pereira PN, Nakajima M, Tagami J, Pashley DH. Long-term durability of resin dentin interface: nanoleakage vs. microtensile bond strength. Oper Dent 2002; 27:289–296.

Paul SJ, Welter DA, Ghazi M, Pashley D. Nanoleakage at the dentin adhesive interface vs microtensile bond strength. Oper Dent 1999; 24:181–188.

Patel DK, Burke FJ. Fractures of posterior teeth: a review and analysis of associated factors. Prim Dent Care 1995; 2:6–10.

Poulsen P. Retention of glass ionomer sealant in primary teeth in young children. Eur J Paediatr Dent 2003; 4:96–98.

Van Dijken JW. Direct resin composite inlays/onlays: an 11 year follow-up. J Dent 2000; 28:299–306.

Van Nieuwenhuysen JP, D'Hoore W, Carvalho J, Qvist V. Long-term evaluation of extensive restorations in permanent teeth. J Dent 2003; 31:395–405.

Wilson NH, Wilson MA, Wastell DG, Smith GA Performance of occlusin in butt-joint and bevel-edged preparations: five-year results. Dent Mater 1991; 7:92–98.

4 The Single Crown, Veneers, and Bleaching

Crowns, veneers, and bleaching of teeth aim to improve the appearance of the patient and are often considered together when discussing the treatment options with patients.

4.1
The Single Crown

When considering the planning of a single-veneer crown, one might start by considering the different ways that the crown might fail in the future. There has been a recent decline in the use of cast gold restorations because of the poor esthetics of this material, although cast gold restorations can have excellent longevity (Donovan et al. 2004).

4.1.1
Recurrent Caries and Periodontal Disease

The patient must have satisfactory oral hygiene before commencing tooth preparation for advanced restorative procedures, otherwise failure is inevitable. The teeth should be examined and the extent of caries and existing restorations noted. The plaque accumulation in the stagnation area around an interproximal caries lesion is often associated with gingivitis (Fig. 4.1). Placing a well-contoured temporary restoration to resolve the gingival inflammation is often a necessary first step (Fig. 4.2). The tooth should undergo a thorough visual examination (Fig. 4.3). A radiographic examination is necessary to ascertain the extent of recurrent caries prior to crown preparation (Fig. 4.4).

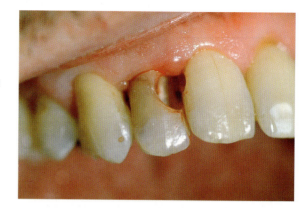

Fig. 4.1 Routine operative dentistry should always be completed prior to advanced procedures. Operative intervention allows the assessment of the extent of caries prior to crown preparation

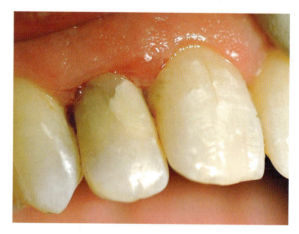

Fig. 4.2 Interproximal caries lesion may be associated with gingivitis, and a well-contoured temporary restoration can allow healing. This facilitates impression taking for crowns and allows careful planning of the crown margin

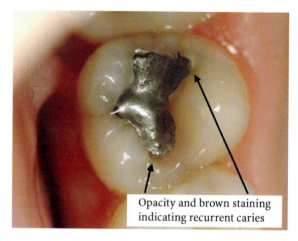

Fig. 4.3 A periapical radiograph is essential prior to crown preparation to assess the periodontal bone support, root length, and the extent of caries, if present. However, radiography underestimates the extent of caries

Opacity and brown staining indicating recurrent caries

4.1 The Single Crown

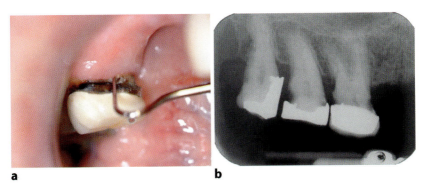

Fig. 4.4 (a) Could this carious cavity on the upper right first molar be repaired with a simple restoration, or would the metal-ceramic crown require replacement? (b) A radiograph revealed that extensive caries was present on the distal interproximal surface, and the metal-ceramic crown therefore required replacement

4.1.2
The Tooth Becomes Nonvital

Unfortunately, about 4–8% of crowned teeth become nonvital in the first 10 years following tooth preparation. A further unknown percentage was probably nonvital before crown preparation of the tooth began, but this can be avoided by assessing the tooth clinically and radiographically. Swelling or erythema of the apical tissues, fistulae, and a tooth that is tender to percussion are all indicative of an endodontic complication that requires further investigation. A prolonged patient response with thermal tests such as ethyl chloride applied on a pledget of cotton wool or warm gutta percha is indicative of irreversible pulpitis. The water spray coolant must be directed to the bur during crown preparation, to prevent overheating of the tooth and pulpal necrosis.

4.1.3
The Crown Restoration Becomes Loose

One of the common reasons for a single veneer crown becoming loose is that the conventional cement lute fails because of repeated loading in tension, especially if the patient has severe parafunctional habits. Most traditional cements are brittle, strong in compression but weak in tension, and are easily damaged by flexing of a thin metal casting. For metal-ceramic crowns, a minimum metal thickness of 0.2 mm is required for base-metal alloys and 0.5 mm for gold alloys. The modern adhesive resin cements are less susceptible to this mode of failure and have the advantage of improved retention of crowns with overtapered preparations.

Single crowns require planning using casts mounted on a semiadjustable articulator with the aid of a facebow recording. Using shimstock, the patient's intraoral occlusal contacts should be compared with those of the mounted casts. Small differences can be corrected on the mounted casts by careful trimming of the occlusal surfaces, whereas larger differences require the casts be rearticulated.

Good adaptation of a gold veneer crown to the prepared tooth surface can be prevented if spicules of cast metal are preventing adequate seating of the restoration. More subtle discrepancies can be corrected by coating the fitting surface with a disclosing dye and pressing the crown onto the tooth. The discrepant areas shine through the dye (Fig. 4.5).

Marking the dynamic and centric occlusion of the natural teeth with articulating paper provides information that may be useful in designing the final restoration. Where the dentist is providing a single unit restoration with teeth on either side, the patient's resulting occlusion should aim to conform to the existing occlusion. Therefore, when moving the jaw laterally with the teeth together, the ideal dynamic occlusion occurs when only the anterior teeth guide the movement of the mandible and the posterior teeth are not in contact. If nonworking-side, premature contacts occur with the final restoration, then unpleasant sequelae can result because of the damag-

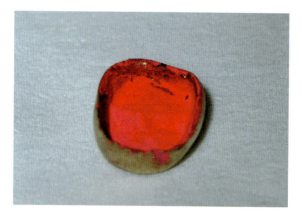

Fig. 4.5 Small discrepant areas of tight contact of the crown with the tooth can be localized using a disclosing dye that is applied to the fitting surface of the crown. The crown is pressed into place and discrepant areas are visible where the metal shines through the dye layer

4.1 The Single Crown

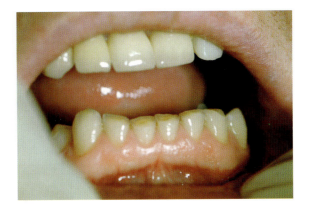

Fig. 4.6 Wear of the lower incisor teeth was caused by the upper porcelain crowns. Replacement of the crowns with metal-ceramic crowns is indicated to provide a less abrasive metal palatal surface

ing horizontal loading on the teeth; the restoration can become uncemented, the tooth may become painful, or temporomandibular joint disorders can result.

In restorations with a porcelain occlusal or incisal surface, occlusal adjustment at the chairside produces an abrasive surface, which if left unpolished will cause wear of the opposing teeth (Fig. 4.6). Where occlusal adjustment of a porcelain restoration is thought likely, it can be tried in at the bisque stage, adjusted, and then glazed. Occlusal marking on glazed porcelain or highly polished metal surfaces can be difficult to see, especially if the teeth are moist. Bausch (Köln, Germany) manufacture a range of thicknesses of articulating test films with an emulsifier that allows the color marking of moist occlusal surfaces. Marking the occlusal contacts of the tooth with the blue, 200-μm-thick articulating paper provides a background against which the finer, red 8-μm-thick film can be used. The second red articulating film contacts are easily seen against the blue background. Thin articulating paper is essential to produce definite occlusal contacts and avoid producing inaccurate smeared contacts.

Adequate retention of a full-veneer gold crown on a molar requires adequate height to the preparation, about 4 mm, given a typical convergence of opposing axial walls of 10–20°. Overtapering the distal surface of an upper crown preparation is a common error as direct vision is not often possible (Fig. 4.7). Where a crown has previously failed because the preparation was too tapered, the preparation can be modified to form multiple steps, rather than creating a very wide margin. Grooves, made parallel to the path of insertion of the crown, also increase retention. Overpreparation in the axial plane with a torpedo-shaped bur results in an unsatisfactory marginal "lip" (Fig. 4.8).

Fig. 4.7 Producing a crown preparation with ideal convergence of opposing axial walls of 10–20° is difficult. In this example, the total convergence is greater (30°), caused by overtapering the distal axial wall of the preparation

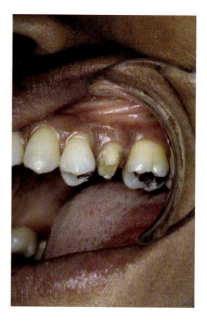

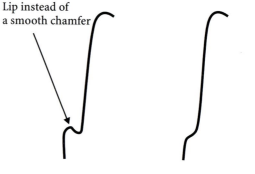

Fig. 4.8 Overpreparation in the axial plane with a torpedo-shaped bur results in an unsatisfactory marginal "lip"

The resistance of the tooth to displacing forces is determined by the taper, height, and width of the preparation. In addition, the maintenance of inclines on the occlusal surface of the preparation, or creation of an occlusal isthmus, can increase resistance to occlusal forces. The luting cement used to attach the crown to the tooth influences the retention of the crown, and must also resist the cyclic masticatory loading. There are many different types of cement available to the dentist, such as zinc phosphate, glass ionomer, zinc polycarboxylate, or reinforced zinc oxide-eugenol, but they lack significant

4.1 The Single Crown

Fig. 4.9 Preserving the mesial wall of enamel in this crown preparation has resulted in a crown with reduced retention

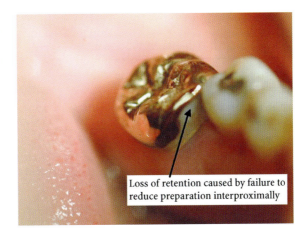

Loss of retention caused by failure to reduce preparation interproximally

adhesion to the teeth and are soluble. Glass ionomer cements release fluoride and therefore prevent recurrent caries around the crown. The new resin-based luting systems can bond to the tooth, have superior mechanical properties, are insoluble, and have reduced microleakage.

The three-quarter crown does not have as favorable a longevity as the full-veneer crown, probably because it lacks the retention of the latter restoration. (Fig. 4.9).

4.1.4
Perforation of the Crown During Occlusal Adjustment

This occurs most commonly as a result of insufficient preparation (Fig. 4.10), for example of the functional cusp bevel on the centric cusp. It is recognized

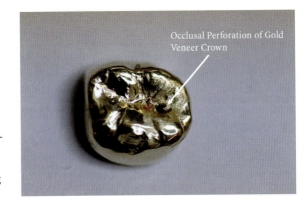

Occlusal Perforation of Gold Veneer Crown

Fig. 4.10 Insufficient reduction of the preparation has resulted in perforation of the full gold crown during placement

Table 4.1 Posterior and anterior crown preparations

Posterior crown preparation				
	Occlusal reduction	Facial reduction	Lingual reduction	Gingival finish
Porcelain fused to metal	1.5–2 mm for metal and porcelain	1.5 mm	0.7-mm-wide chamfer	0.3-mm-wide gingival bevel
Full-veneer metal crown	1 mm on functional cusp 1.5 mm on nonfunctional cusp	Occurs in two planes	Occurs in two planes	1-mm-wide chamfer

Anterior crown preparation				
	Occlusal reduction	Facial reduction	Lingual reduction	Gingival finish
Porcelain fused to metal	2-mm incisal reduction	1.2 mm reduction	0.7 mm if metal*	0.5-mm-wide chamfer

* The metal/porcelain junction must not be in direct occlusal contact in centric occlusion

by the occlusal surface being too wide following occlusal reduction, with the cusp tips of the preparation not in line with the cusps of the other teeth in the arch. Preparing the functional cusp bevel returns the centric cusp tip into line with the other teeth in the arch. The functional cusp bevel is prepared at 30–45° to the vertical, parallel to the opposing cusp inclination. The lingual axial reduction must also allow a natural lingual contour to be established; therefore the occlusal quarter of the tooth is reduced at 30–45°. Insufficient preparation results in the technician producing an occlusal interference in an attempt to produce a crown of sufficient thickness (see Table 4.1).

4.1.5
The Appearance of the Crown is Unsatisfactory

Many crowns are unsatisfactory because they appear too different from the other teeth around them. This can be a result of poor shade matching or an incorrect shape to the teeth.

4.1.5.1
Shade of the Crown

The standard porcelain shade guide is the Vitapan guide, which has A shades with a red-brown hue, and B shades with a yellow hue. Each hue is further subdivided into increasing chroma. The D range represents a lower value (dark–light) of the A range, whereas the C range represents a lower value of the B range. Crowns are often unsatisfactory because they are too high in value in relation to the surrounding teeth, appearing white, opaque, and "lifeless". Inadequate tooth reduction will allow the opaque porcelain or metal to become apparent.

Shade taking is handicapped by the inadequacy of some shade guides and the limited range of some of the ceramic shades that are available. For metal-ceramic crowns, the type of metal and porcelain used, the conditions used for firing the porcelain, and the number of firings can have some effect on the final crown restoration color. Gold and palladium alloys can cause a significant yellow shift to the metal-ceramic color compared to the base-metal alloys such as nickel-chrome and cobalt-chromium alloys (Kourtis et al. 2004). An opaque porcelain layer of minimum thickness 0.3 mm will obscure the metal layer underneath (Terada et al. 1989), but the thickness of overlying porcelain required to obscure the opaque layer will vary according to the shade being used. An insufficient thickness of opaque porcelain will allow a gray show-through of the metal. Ideally, individually constructed all-ceramic or metal-ceramic shade guides should be considered. Shade-taking is further complicated by a variable gingival shade, such as with racial pigmentation. Gingivae around crowns are sometimes discolored (have a lower value and chroma) from previous restorations, compared with the gingivae surrounding natural teeth (Takeda et al. 1996), due to their incorporation of metal ion corrosion products.

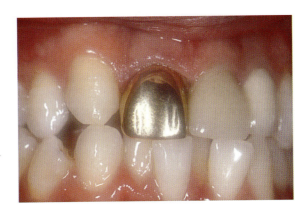

Fig. 4.11 A gold-veneer crown placed on the upper central incisor tooth

Some patients request the prominent show of gold in their anterior teeth (Fig. 4.11). If there is a clinical indication for this material to be used, then there is no reason not to accede to this request. However, if the tooth is healthy and normal then the risks to the tooth associated with crown preparation (such as loss of vitality or fracture, for example) must be explained to the patient before they exercise their judgment whether to proceed.

4.1.5.2
Shape of the Crown

The appearance of the line angle of the tooth gives the best visual cue to the apparent width of the tooth. The line angle, which divides the facial from the interproximal surfaces, must be angled correctly; if they are too close together, the tooth appears narrow. Similarly, placing the line angles far apart causes the tooth to appear wide. The interproximal contact of the central incisors is at the incisal third of the tooth (not at the incisal edge), and the proximal contacts move apically when progressing distally in the arch. Viewed from the buccal aspect, all posterior teeth have their interproximal contacts in the middle third of the tooth, but further posteriorly in the arch the proximal contacts move more cervical in the middle third.

4.1.5.3
Gingival Contour

An underprepared tooth often results in an overcontoured restoration as the technician seeks to create a restoration with sufficient marginal bulk and rigidity. The term "emergence profile" has been used to describe the angle that the outer margin of the crown forms with the tooth root at the gingival sulcus. In the past there has been much emphasis placed on the emergence profile of crowns in the mistaken belief that the crown protects the gingival marginal tissues from abrasive food during mastication. Where meticulous plaque control is maintained and the margins of crowns are placed in a slightly supragingival position, then the periodontal health of the teeth is most likely to be good.

4.1.5.4
Gingival Recession

Teeth with thin marginal gingivae are most prone to gingival recession, exposing the margins of crowns. Trauma to the tissues during tooth preparation

4.1 The Single Crown

must be avoided and placement of crown margins should be at the gingival crest or limited to a depth of 0.5 mm intracrevicular placement. If the margins of a crown preparation are extended onto the root surface and encroach on the the connective tissue attachment of the tooth to the alveolar bone, then repair involves epithelial migration, pocket formation, and subsequent reestablishment of a "biological width" by chronic inflammation and bone resorption. The biological width is a 2-mm-wide region between the base of the gingival sulcus and the alveolar crest, and consists of connective tissue and epithelial attachments.

Electrosurgery to control gingival bleeding must be performed judiciously. The placement of a retraction cord prior to taking impressions for crowns can induce bleeding. Mechanical retraction of the gingival sulcus can be frustratingly difficult as the cord often pops out during placement. When traumatic tooth preparation is combined with the forceful application of hemostatic cord, which is impregnated with astringent solutions, for longer than a few minutes, then gingival recession is inevitable. Extensive gingival necrosis and recession encroaching on the biological width can result (Fig. 4.12).

Where the gingival margins of crowns are subgingivally placed, they can be difficult to record accurately (Fig. 4.13a). Newer methods of gingival sulcus retraction are available that avoid hemostatic agents. Safer, effective gingival retraction is possible using an expanding polyvinylsiloxane material (Magic Foam Cord, Coltene-Whaledent), which is injected around the gingival sulcus and held in place with a shaped cotton pad (Comprecap Anatomic) placed over the tooth. The patient bites gently on the Comprecap Anatomic for 5 min as the material expands and gently retracts the gingiva (Fig. 4.13b). The Comprecap Anatomic is easily removed to reveal a fully retracted gingival sulcus (Fig. 4.13c).

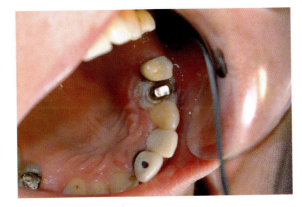

Fig. 4.12 Traumatic tooth preparation, excessive cauterization or prolonged application of hemostatic cord and astringent solutions can cause extensive gingival necrosis

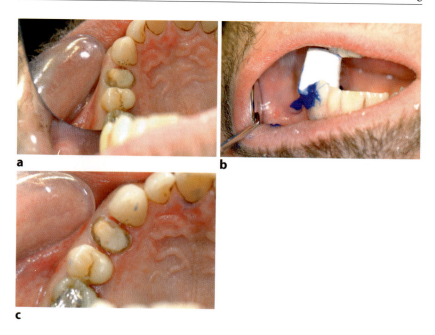

Fig. 4.13 (a) Where bleeding, debris, or gingival exudate is present, subgingival margins are difficult to record accurately using hydrophobic impression materials (such as addition silicones). (b) A blue, expanding polyvinylsiloxane material is injected around the gingival sulcus and held in place with a shaped cotton pad (Comprecap Anatomic) placed over the tooth. The material expands and gently retracts the gingiva. (c) When the cotton pad is removed, a fully retracted gingival sulcus can be seen

4.2
New Developments in Crown Provision

After several crown preparations and the insult from caries, teeth often approach the end of their treatment cycle lacking a retentive coronal tooth structure. Pins can be used on posterior teeth to retain a core such as amalgam, but they may perforate the pulp or periodontal ligament and cause microcracks in an already weakened tooth. Elective devitalization of the tooth and the fitting of a post and core are possible, but this necessitates further tooth removal. Post and core restorations have a poor prognosis where endodontic therapy has caused problems such as excessive tapering of the root canal and perforation of the root canal. With severe endodontic complications, consideration should be given to extracting the tooth and providing an implant-retained crown, which research has shown to be very successful.

Sandblasting the fitting surface of nonprecious and precious metal onlays, and porcelain crowns increases the surface area of their fitting surface so that adhesive bonding with composite resin/dentin bonding agents is possible. In addition, oxidizing or tin-plating gold surfaces will allow them to be bonded to enamel and dentin. Resin-based luting agents are likely to supercede the traditional cements because of their ability to bond the restoration to the tooth. In addition, most of these luting agents are supplied in a range of shades, which makes them much more acceptable for luting esthetic indirect restorations.

Composite-resin luting cements and dentin-bonding agents provide an opportunity to restore teeth that lack the opposing, near-parallel surfaces required for retention of traditional crowns. For traditional crown preparation it was always assumed that cements would be used that lacked adhesion to tooth and crown, and which relied on frictional resistance between crown and tooth. The latest resin-composite luting cements have excellent physical properties, set by autopolymerizing or dual-cure mechanisms, and bond to both the restoration and the tooth. One example of these cements is RelyX Unicem (3M ESPE, Seefeld, Germany), which has a proven clinical record in bonding indirect restorations to dentin. However, it has a low bond strength to enamel unless a separate etching step occurs using a conventional phosphoric acid conditioner.

4.3
Veneers

Porcelain laminate veneers are becoming popular because they restore the esthetics of a tooth with minimal tooth preparation (Walls et al. 2002). Some tooth preparation is absolutely essential, as optimal retention requires that the aprismatic surface enamel be removed. However, most of the studies that have reported on the success of these restorations have been only short-term, less than 5 years.

It is always advisable to examine the occlusion before tooth preparation. Will the veneer be protected in lateral movements by contact with other teeth? Veneers are generally contraindicated where the patient has bruxist parafunctional habits.

4.3.1
Tooth Preparation

Opinion is divided as to the optimal preparation design for veneers, but there is little published evidence to allow a rational recommendation to be made

(Fig. 4.14). Several studies report that incisal edge coverage with porcelain provides a better result. With a beveled incisal edge or more extensive overlap design, the incisal edge is replaced in porcelain. Covering the incisal edge in porcelain can provide an esthetic, translucent edge (Fig. 4.15). It becomes easier to seat the restoration during cementation procedures, as there is a definite stop, and the resulting improved adaptation of the veneer avoids marginal discrepancies and staining. A chamfer finish line on the gingival and proximal surfaces will preserve the enamel in the marginal regions to allow optimal adhesive bonding of the veneer. A round-end tapered diamond will provide the correct chamfer shape. The labial surface should be reduced in two planes, with a reduction of about 0.3 mm at the gingiva and 0.5 mm nearer the incisal edge. The preparation must extend into the proximal surface to conceal the restoration margins, but the contact point with the adjacent teeth is preserved. There should be no undercuts and smooth internal line angles.

Retention of veneers is excellent where they cover enamel, but failure of laminate veneers is common where they partially cover preexisting restorations (Shaini et al. 1997). Marginal leakage is then common at the interface of the veneer and the preexisting composite resin. Veneers are also used inappropriately where they are used to cover extensive class IV composite

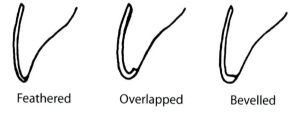

Fig. 4.14 The three main types of veneer preparation that are used

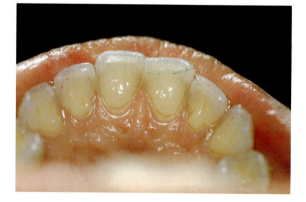

Fig. 4.15 With the more extensive beveled or overlapped preparation designs, an esthetic, translucent incisal edge in porcelain can be produced

restorations. Veneers are contraindicated if the remaining tooth surface is less than 50% enamel. In such situations, a full coverage crown would be a more durable option.

4.3.2
Disadvantages of Veneers

Veneers provide an excellent esthetic result, but are also used inappropriately, in some cases, to provide "quick-fix" orthodontics, by correcting quite extensive malocclusions. As a result of providing veneers, the labial surfaces of the teeth are aligned, but the teeth may be bulky and unesthetic, with thick incisal edges and an incorrect emergence profile to the gingival surface. Extensive tooth preparation is usually required, with the result that the veneer must adhere to a periphery of dentin, not enamel, with a consequent reduction in veneer retention. Adequate hardening of the resin cement is reduced when using thick porcelain veneers (greater than 0.7 mm), as they reduce the light transmission during polymerization. Dual-cure resin cements are essential for the bonding of thick veneers.

Anterior veneers obtain their fracture resistance from the adhesive bond to the underlying tooth surface. There is little advantage, therefore, in using high-strength veneer porcelains as an increased material strength is unnecessary in this situation. Fortress (Mirage Dental Systems, KS, USA) is a leucite-reinforced, high-strength porcelain that can be etched and bonded to the teeth. However, the uniformly homogenous dispersal of 3- to 4-µm-diameter leucite particles in Fortress does make this material a low abrasive ceramic with excellent esthetics.

4.3.3
Failure of Veneers

Porcelain veneers are successful esthetic restorations (see Table 4.2). Figure 4.16 illustrates the veneer restoration of the two upper central incisor teeth. Peumans et al. (1998) showed that 93% of restorations were excellent after 5 years, while failures were due to recurrent caries, fracture, microleakage, or a pulpal reaction. Studies have shown that veneers do suffer large marginal gaps, probably due to poor location of the veneer onto the tooth during cementation and wear of the resin luting cement (Peumans et al. 2000). Marginal discrepancies may also occur due to the polymerization shrinkage of the luting resin cement. This can be minimized by using a highly filled resin. The commercially available luting cements differ considerably in their filler loading. Dentin exposure is inevitable in some cases, but the inability

Table 4.2 Summary table of success rate of veneers

Dumfahrt and Schaffer (2000)	91% Estimated survival at 10 years
Dunne and Millar (1993)	89% Survival up to 63 months
Kreulen et al. (1998)	92% Survival after 3 years
Peumans et al. (1998)	93% Success rate after 5 years

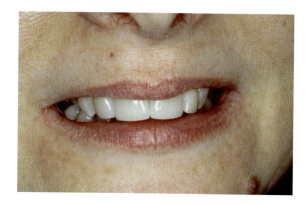

Fig. 4.16 This patient's smile has been transformed by the porcelain veneers replacing the upper central incisor teeth

of current dentin bonding agents to hermetically seal the veneer margin can lead to microleakage in the long term.

Given the less than perfect long-term success rate of veneers, improving the shade of teeth should first be undertaken using bleaching techniques. Veneers, although requiring minimal intervention, often require crowns when they fail. Restoring a single, discolored tooth with an esthetic veneer is most challenging. The thin porcelain layer of the veneer has to perform two conflicting functions; it must prevent the dark tooth underneath showing through and yet still provide a translucent appearance. Using a conventional crown instead, with its greater tooth reduction, allows an opaque porcelain to be used with overlying dentin and translucent porcelains.

Silane assists in bonding the resin cement to the etched porcelain, but it has a limited shelf life (about 1 year) and quickly undergoes decomposition if left unrefridgerated. The silane forms siloxane bonds (Si-O-Si) that bind it to the ceramic surface, and also bonds with the methacrylate groups of the resin. The hydrolysis of the silane may be responsible for the gradual degradation of the bond strength between ceramic and resin.

Freehand preparation often causes overpreparation of the enamel in the cervical area of the teeth (Nattress et al. 1995), but depth gauge burs (e.g., Brasseler Laminate Veneer System Set 4151, Brasseler, USA, Savannah, GA,

USA) and depth grooves can reduce the likelihood of this occurring. The facial enamel is usually reduced by 0.3–0.5 mm, but where the underlying tooth is severely discolored, reduction should be 0.7 mm. After discussion with the patient, both dentist and patient may decide that tooth preparation without anesthesia will allow determination of whether dentin has been exposed or not. Where dentin has been exposed during tooth preparation, it must be protected with a primer or desensitizing agent prior to dismissing the patient. This avoids postoperative sensitivity with cold fluids and has no deleterious effect on the retention of the final veneer restoration. The margin of the preparation should be placed at the gingival crest or slightly subgingival, but always trying to ensure a margin in enamel.

4.3.4
Cementation Procedures for a Veneer

Cementation procedures require that the fragile veneer be handled gently. Adjustments other than to interproximal contacts to allow seating of the restoration should be carried out after cementation is complete. The inner surface of the veneer is etched in the laboratory. Try-in pastes can be used to modify the shade of the veneer and are removed with acetone after the trial insertion. While the dentist is preparing the tooth, the dental assistant coats the intaglio surface of the veneer with silane, which is allowed to dry, and then applies a thin layer of unfilled resin. The dentist cleans the tooth with pumice paste and applies plastic matrices to the interproximal contacts of the teeth. The tooth is etched with phosphoric acid gel for 20 s, washed for 20 s, and then the enamel is dried to the typical frosty white appearance. The primer/bonding resins are applied to the tooth and light-cured for 90 s.

The resin composite is applied to the veneer, which is pressed gently into place. Light polymerization over the central area of the veneer for 10 s will allow the veneer to be held in place while a small sable brush moistened with bonding resin can be used to remove excess unset cement at the margin. This avoids dragging the cement from underneath the veneer and thereby prevents creation of a marginal deficiency (Tay et al. 1987). The resin cement is further cured for 30 s each from the lingual and facial aspects. Excess cement can be removed with a fine carbide bur and composite polishing points.

4.3.5
Provisional Restorations for Veneers

In situations where a patient requests a temporary, esthetic restoration while the veneer is being manufactured, then a small area of the labial surface of the tooth (about 2 mm²) can be etched, and a small quantity of unfilled resin applied and cured. Composite resin can be applied in a thin layer over the whole labial surface of the tooth and light-cured for 20 s. Maidment (1999) described an indirect technique in which a registration is taken of the tooth prior to tooth preparation, using a transparent silicone material (Memosil CD, manufactured by Heraeus Kulzer, Armonk, NY, USA). After the veneer preparation is complete, the registration is filled with composite resin and placed back on the tooth. The composite resin is light cured for 40 s through the transparent registration material and then again for a further 20 s when it has been retrieved from the patient's mouth. The temporary veneer is then attached to a small area of etched tooth enamel using light-cured resin. The manufacturers also recommend the use of the transparent registration material Memosil CD when fabricating provisional crowns and bridges.

4.4
Resin-Bonded All-Ceramic Crowns (or "Dentin-Bonded Crown")

The resin-bonded all-ceramic crown is essentially a veneer that has extended to include full coverage of the tooth crown. The technique has found application in treating bulimic patients with severe tooth erosion (Milosevic and Jones 1996) and in the treatment of patients with amelogenesis imperfecta (Fig. 4.17). In both situations, preserving the maximum amount of remaining tooth in the young patient is an essential requirement if the tooth is to have a long-term survival. Porcelain is bonded to the prepared tooth surface using a dentin-bonding agent and a dual-cure, resin-composite luting cement. The porcelain restoration is essentially fragile, but gains its strength from the adhesive bond with the tooth. Low-fusing feldspathic porcelain,

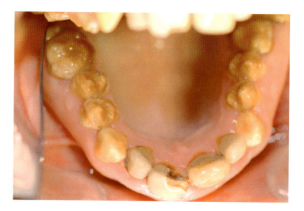

Fig. 4.17 This patient has the genetic condition amelogenesis imperfecta, which has resulted in the absence of formation of enamel on her teeth

4.4 Resin-Bonded All-Ceramic Crowns (or "Dentin-Bonded Crown")

leucite-reinforced porcelain, and pressed-glass ceramics are suitable for this application. Fortress (Chameleon Dental, KS, USA) is a leucite-reinforced ceramic material with enhanced fracture resistance over feldspathic porcelain crowns. Burke (1999) showed that fracture of Fortress crowns under compressive loading tended to protect the underlying tooth from damage, allowing restoration of the tooth with a new crown.

The preparation for resin bonded all-ceramic crowns involves:

1. Supragingival placement of margins. This is important to avoid subsequent microleakage. With subgingival placement of margins, moisture control is difficult, resulting in poor adhesion to cementum and dentin. Where esthetics dictates that a subgingival preparation is essential, then a conventionally designed crown is indicated. Preservation of enamel at the margin of the resin-bonded all-ceramic crown preparation provides an optimal bond.
2. Rounded line angles to reduce stress concentration in the ceramic. This allows good adaptation of the restoration to the tooth.
3. A chamfer margin allows a clearly visible finishing line for the technician without the margin of the restoration appearing too thin and fragile. The gingival response to the porcelain surface is usually excellent.

Resin-bonded all-ceramic crown preparations of upper central incisor teeth are illustrated in Fig. 4.18. Because retention of resin-bonded all-ceramic crowns is dependent on enamel and dentin adhesion, factors such as the height of the preparation and preparation taper are not as critical as with conventional crowns. Despite the minimal preparation and the relatively thin layer of porcelain that is utilized, these crowns have a good fracture resistance, provided a dentin-bonding system rather than conventional cement is used.

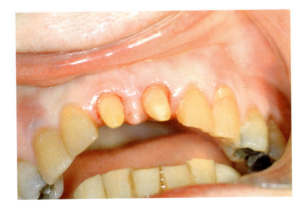

Fig. 4.18 Preparations for resin-bonded ceramic crowns should be rounded, with a chamfer margin placed supragingivally where possible

Where there has been a core buildup to replace missing tooth substance, retention and support for a dentin-bonded crown is therefore reduced. The in vitro fracture resistance of teeth with dentin-bonded ceramic crowns is higher with a pinned amalgam core than using a relatively weak core material such as glass ionomer (Lang et al. 2003).

4.4.1
Marginal Leakage

Marginal leakage at the cervical margins of single-unit all-porcelain crowns is a common finding. In-vitro studies report that 60–80% of restorations undergo leakage where the margin is placed on dentin below the cementoenamel junction (Ferrari et al. 1999).

4.4.2
Cementation Procedures for the Resin-Bonded All-Ceramic Crown

A dentin-bonding agent should be used that provides minimal film thickness combined with a dual-cure, resin-composite luting system. Variolink II (Ivoclar Vivodent) is a suitable dual-cure resin cement with a film thickness of only 22 µm. The low viscosity catalyst has a filler content of 71% by weight. This particular system has a range of try-in pastes that match the corresponding six shades of base luting cement, although with any luting system, the degree of change in the crown shade that can be obtained is limited. The esthetic result obtained with resin-bonded all-ceramic crowns is acceptable and usually superior to that obtained with metal-ceramic crowns. This is because the resin cement is translucent, allowing light to reflect naturally from the dentin beneath. When an enamel and dentin conditioning, universal bonding agent (such as Etch and Prime 3.0) is used with Variolink II, it has been shown that excellent marginal adaptation of the porcelain is possible (Clotten et al. 1999). This can be attributed to the simplified technique.

Where the fitting surface of the crown has been sandblasted, 35% phosphoric acid should be applied to that surface for 30 s, then washed off and dried. This acid does not etch the porcelain surface but merely provides a cleaner surface. The all-ceramic crown is etched with hydrofluoric acid to create a roughened intaglio surface. A silane bonding agent should then be applied to the crown fitting surface for 1 min to enhance the bond strength of the resin cement to the porcelain. The tooth is etched and a primer and dual-cured adhesive applied. Adhesive resin is also applied to the fitting surface of the crown. The dual-cure luting material is applied to the fitting surface of the crown. The crown is seated gently, and excess material removed from the crown margins prior to light-curing. The resin cement should be cured for 1 min each from the labial and palatal aspects.

One major disadvantage of the resin-bonded all-ceramic crown is that the occlusion can only be checked after the restoration has been finally luted into position. Another disadvantage is that no long-term studies are available to assess the likelihood of failure of these restorations in comparison to more traditional forms of treatment. Short-term studies, such as that by Burke et al. (2001), showed that after 1 year, 90 of the 98 available restorations were intact and satisfactory – a success rate of nearly 92%. The main reason for failure was fracture in six crowns and cracking of a further two.

4.5
Bleaching of Teeth

The successful bleaching of unsightly, dark teeth can be very satisfying for the dentist and patient. It is a safe procedure with few side effects, and is much less invasive than other techniques such as veneering or crowning of teeth, which require tooth preparation. Problems associated with bleaching, for example sensitivity of the teeth and gingival ulceration, are more common when higher concentrations of bleaching agents have been used. Staining of teeth caused by tetracycline tends to be resistant to bleaching, whereas the yellowing of teeth as a result of age is often very successfully treated. The gray staining of enamel caused by amalgam corrosion cannot be removed by bleaching solutions. Bleaching is generally successful, but the whitened appearance of the teeth seldom lasts more than several years.

4.5.1
Cervical Resorption

More serious side effects such as external root resorption may occur when a higher than 30% concentration of hydrogen peroxide is used in combination with heat (as in the thermocatalytic technique). Hydroxyl groups may be generated during thermocatalytic bleaching, especially where ethylenediaminetetraacetic acid has been used previously to clean the tooth. Hydroxyl ions may stimulate cells in the cervical periodontal ligament to differentiate into odontoclasts, which begin root resorption in the area of the tooth below the epithelial attachment (Dahlstrom et al. 1997).

Cervical resorption is usually painless until the resorption exposes the pulp, necessitating endodontic therapy. Intracanal dressings of calcium hydroxide are often successful in halting further tooth resorption, but severe external root resorption often necessitates extraction of the tooth. Moderate root resorption can be treated by orthodontically extruding the tooth and restoring it with a post-retained crown, but the prognosis of this treatment can be doubtful. Mild cervical resorption can be treated by surgical access, curettage, and placement of a restoration.

4.5.2
The "Walking Bleach" Technique

In this procedure the dentist seals a paste of sodium perborate into the pulp chamber of a discolored nonvital tooth, such as the maxillary central incisor illustrated in Fig. 4.19. Bleaching produces an excellent result in most cases. The technique is safe as only a low concentration of hydrogen peroxide (about 3%) is released. A study by Holmstrup et al. (1998) of 95 teeth examined 3 years after treatment with sodium perborate and water showed no signs of cervical root resorption. Higher concentrations of hydrogen peroxide should not be used either alone or mixed with sodium perborate, as the prolonged contact is likely to cause cervical root resorption. Nonvital teeth often become discolored as a result of pulp tissue and blood degradation, which form dark products that are retained by the dentin. Colored molecules, such as ferric sulphide, are reduced by the radicals formed during the decomposition of hydrogen peroxide and are converted to colorless ferrous compounds.

A radiographic check of the status of the periapical seal must be undertaken prior to application of any bleaching medicaments. This is to ensure that a well-condensed root filling is in situ, and that the bleaching agent will not reach the apical tissues and cause damage. The tooth is isolated with a rubber dam and a lingual access cavity is prepared into the pulp chamber. Any pulpal

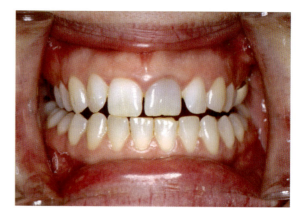

Fig. 4.19 In the "walking bleach method," sodium perborate is placed into the pulp chamber of a discolored nonvital tooth

remnants, previous restorative materials, or root filling materials are removed to a depth of 2 mm below the enamel-cementum junction.

A protective layer of glass ionomer cement is placed into the root canal to prevent diffusion of the hydrogen peroxide through the dentin to the periodontium where it may initiate cervical root resorption. In the interproximal area of the anterior teeth, the epithelial attachment rises incisally so the intracoronal barrier must also follow this curve. The glass ionomer cement barrier must extend about 1 mm incisal to the cementoenamel junction. The bleaching agent paste (sodium perborate mixed with distilled water) is applied to the pulp chamber and condensed into place. The bleaching agent must remain in place for about 4 days, which requires that a retentive, temporary polycarboxylate restoration be used. Several reapplications of the sodium perborate mixture may be necessary until a satisfactory color is achieved.

Composite resins have a reduced adhesion to bleached enamel and dentin, because the increased oxygen content of the dental tissues inhibits polymerization of the resin. In addition, the pH of the dentin surface is raised (Elkhatib et al. 2003). Remaining hydrogen-peroxide-containing medicaments can be removed by applying a pretreatment solution of sodium hypochlorite, followed by cleaning and dehydrating the enamel with alcohol. It is difficult to predict the final shade with any bleaching technique. The color of composite resin restorations is unaffected by the bleaching agent, so final restorations should be placed after the tooth bleaching has taken place.

4.5.3
Vital Tooth Bleaching

The most popular method for bleaching vital teeth uses a custom-made plastic tray that the patient uses to apply a 10% solution of carbamide peroxide to their teeth overnight for about 2 weeks. The American Dental Association approves the use of 10% carbamide peroxide (pH 7) in trays for home use. This concentration of carbamide peroxide is equivalent to about 3% hydrogen peroxide, but is safe despite a large percentage being ingested (Dahl and Pallesen 2003). Higher concentrations of 10%, 15%, 20%, 35%, and 38% carbamide peroxide are commercially available (Optident, Ilkley, UK).

Adhesive disposable gel trays containing 9% hydrogen peroxide are also available (Optident), which can be applied by the patient to their teeth for 30–60 min each day.

Many patients complain of tooth sensitivity, which may last for a few days after treatment has finished. Patients can be recommended to use a fluoride mouthwash or desensitizing toothpaste prior to application of the carbamide peroxide gel. The reason for the increased sensitivity of teeth may be due to penetration of the hydrogen peroxide into the pulp where it may damage odontoblasts and cause hemorrhage and inflammation. Mucosal irritation is also a relatively common side effect, but this can be minimized by using a tray that only contacts the teeth and avoids the gingival tissues.

4.5.4
In-House Tooth Bleaching

In-office procedures use 35% hydrogen peroxide applied for 30 min on several separate occasions. At this concentration, hydrogen peroxide is caustic to the gingival tissues, so rubber-dam isolation of the teeth is recommended. Contraindications to the use of hydrogen peroxide at this high concentration include patients with cracks in their teeth or pregnant females.

External prophylaxis of the teeth is first recommended to remove surface staining. The use of local anesthesia should be avoided so that if the patient feels tingling of the gingiva the technique can be abandoned and the area washed with water or a sodium bicarbonate mouthwash. The hydrogen peroxide is applied to the tooth using a cotton bud. Applying heat from a light-curing unit several times during the session increases the speed at which the hydrogen peroxide solution bleaches the tooth.

4.6
Microabrasion

Microabrasion is a technique that can be used by the dentist first, then supplemented with home treatment by the patient using topical carbamide peroxide. The teeth should be isolated with a rubber dam. A slurry of hydrochloric acid mixed with particles of silicon carbide (Opalustre; manufactured by Ultradent, Utah, USA) can remove superficial stains when brushed into the surface of the teeth. Brushes such as the small ICB brushes manufactured by Ultradent are suitable. The patient shown in Fig. 4.20 presented with discolored, hypoplastic anterior teeth and requested the minimum intervention that would remove the brown staining. After discussion with the patient about the different treatment options, the patient requested microabrasion. Microabrasion of the teeth was performed under a rubber dam and the brown staining was removed (Fig. 4.20b). The patient complained of some mild sensitivity to cold drinks following the treatment, which was relieved by successive applications of a thin layer of adhesive fluoride varnish (Fig. 4.20c). Hypoplasia of central incisor teeth is a relatively common occurrence (Fig. 4.21) and may be due to fluorosis, localized infection of an overlying deciduous tooth, or exanthematous fevers in childhood.

4.6 Microabrasion

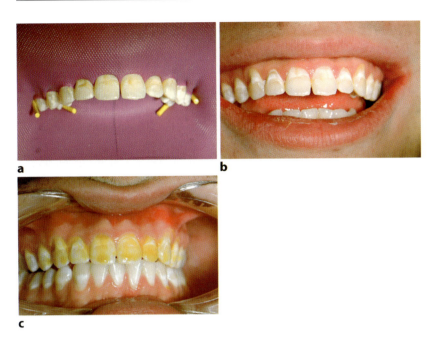

Fig. 4.20 (a) This patient presented with discolored, hypoplastic anterior teeth. (b) Using a rubber dam, a slurry of hydrochloric acid mixed with particles of silicon carbide was brushed onto the teeth and the brown staining was removed. (c) The patient complained of mild tooth sensitivity following microabrasion. This was reduced by applying a thin layer of fluoride varnish to the microabraded teeth

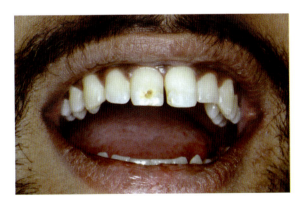

Fig. 4.21 Microabrasion can be used to treat hypoplastic incisors with small localized defects

References

Burke FJ, Hussey DL, McCaughey AD. Evaluation of the 1-year clinical performance of dentin-bond ceramic crowns and four case reports. Quintessence Int 2001; 32:593-601.

Burke FJT. Fracture resistance of teeth restored with dentin-bonded crowns constructed in a leucite-reinforced ceramic. Dent Mater 1999; 15:359-362.

Clotten S, Blunck U, Roulet JF. The influence of a simplified application technique for ceramic inlays on the margin quality. J Adhes Dent 1999; 1:159-166.

Dahl JE, Pallesen U. Tooth bleaching – a critical review of the biological aspects. Crit Rev Biol Med 2003; 14:292-304.

Dahlstrom SW, Heithersay GS, Bridges TE. Hydroxyl radical activity in thermocatalytically bleached root-filled teeth. Endod Dent Traumatol 1997; 13:119-125.

Donovan T, Simonsen RJ, Guertin G, Tucker RV. Retrospective clinical evaluation of 1,314 cast gold restorations in service from 1 to 52 years. J Esthet Restor Dent 2004; 16:194-204.

Dumfahrt H, Schaffer H. Porcelain laminate veneers. A retrospective evaluation after 1 to 10 years of service: Part II–Clinical results. Int J Prosthodont 2000; 13:9-18.

Dunne SM, Millar BJ. A longitudinal study of the clinical performance of porcelain veneers. Br Dent J 1993; 175:317-321.

Elkhatib H, Nakajima M, Hiraishi N, Kitasako Y, Tagami J, Nomura S. Surface pH and bond strength of a self-etching primer/adhesive system to intracoronal dentin after application of hydrogen peroxide bleach with sodium perborate. Oper Dent 2003; 28:591-597.

Ferrari M, Mannocci F, Mason PN, Kugel G. In vitro leakage of resin-bonded all-porcelain crowns. J Adhes Dent 1999; 1:233-242.

Holmstrup G, Palm AM, Lambjerg-Hansen H. Bleaching of discolored root-filled teeth. Endod Dent Traumatol 1988; 4:197-201.

Kourtis SG, Tripodakis AP, Doukoudakis AA. Spectrophotometric evaluation of the optical influence of different metal alloys and porcelains in the metal-ceramic complex. J Prosthet Dent 2004; 92:477-485.

Kreulen CM, Creugers NH, Meijering AC. Meta-analysis of anterior veneer restorations in clinical studies. J Dent 1998; 26:345-353.

Lang M, McHugh S, Burke FJ. In vitro fracture resistance of teeth with dentin-bonded ceramic crowns and core build-ups. Am J Dent 2003; 16 Spec No:88A-96A.

Maidment Y. Provisional restoration of veneer preparations: a modified technique. Dent Update 1999; 26:392-393.

Milosevic A, Jones C. Use of resin-bonded ceramic crowns in a bulimic patient with severe tooth erosion. Quintessence Int 1996; 27:123-127.

Nattress BR, Youngson, CC, Patterson JW, Martin DM, Ralph JP. An in vitro assessment of tooth preparation for porcelain veneer restorations. J Dent 1995; 23:165-170.

Peumans M, Van Meerbeek B, Lambrechts P, Vanherle G. Porcelain veneers: a review of the literature. J Dent 2000; 28:163-177.

Peumans M, Van Meerbeek B, Lambrechts P, Vuylsteke-Wauters M, Vanherle G. Five-year clinical performance of porcelain veneers. Quintessence Int 1998; 29:211-221.

Shaini FJ, Shortall AC, Marquis PM. Higher failure rate associated with veneers over existing restorations. J Oral Rehabil 1997; 24:553-559.

References

Takeda T, Ishigami K, Shimada A, Ohki K. A study of discoloration of the gingiva by artificial crowns. Int J Prosthodont 1996; 9:197–202.

Tay WM, Lynch E, Auger D. Effects of some finishing techniques on cervical margins of porcelain laminates. Quintessence Int 1987; 18:599–602.

Terada, Y; Sakai, T; Hirayasu, R. The masking ability of an opaque porcelain: a spectrophotometric study. Int J Prosthodont 1989; 2:259–264.

Walls AWG, Steele JG, Wassell RW. Crowns and other extra-coronal restorations: porcelain laminate veneers. Br Dent J 2002; 193:73–82.

5 Noncarious Tooth Tissue Loss

5.1
Noncarious Tooth Wear

Noncarious tooth wear is a common problem. Exposed dentin can result from acidic erosion, abrasion, and attrition, but most toothwear has erosion as the dominant etiological factor. Localized anterior toothwear of the upper anterior teeth is often caused by the consumption of erosive carbonated beverages, fruit juices, and citrus fruits. Regurgitated stomach acid in gastroesophageal reflux disease, hiatus hernia, and esophagitis and vomiting in bulimia, alcoholism, and psychosomatic disorders can cause erosive tooth wear of the palatal surfaces of the anterior teeth. Drugs that tend to reduce the amount of saliva in the mouth, such as antidepressants, recreational drugs (LSD and Ecstasy, which is 3,4-methylene-dioxymethamphetamine), and diuretics, also diminish the buffering capacity available to neutralize dietary or stomach acids. Users of Ecstasy commonly complain of a dry mouth, and erosion from carbonated beverages is thought to be an important etiological factor. However, the occlusal surfaces of the molar teeth are more commonly affected than the incisor teeth, which would indicate that jaw clenching and masseter muscle hyperactivity are important (Milosevic et al. 1999). Referral to a medical practitioner may be necessary in cases where a medical condition is important in the etiology of the toothwear (e.g., gastroesophageal reflux; Moazzez et al. 2004). Some medical conditions associated with reduced salivation (e.g., Sjogren's syndrome) can predispose to toothwear.

5.1.1
Clinical Appearance of Erosion

Erosion causes smooth, rounded concavities with soft edges to the buccal and lingual/palatal surfaces of teeth. The facial aspects of maxillary anterior teeth are most commonly affected by noncarious cervical lesions (Young and

Khan 2002). The enamel appears dull and there is often an absence of stain (Howden 1971). The upper anterior teeth often have thinned incisal edges that appear translucent. Amalgam and composite restorations are unaffected by the acid and so stand proud of the tooth surface, but elsewhere on the tooth there may be a reduced occlusal contact with the opposing tooth. Wear is often prominent on nonoccluding surfaces. On the occluding surfaces, attrition and erosion may cause the incisal edges of the lower teeth to have dentin exposed, surrounded by enamel ridges (enamel "cupping").

5.1.2
Clinical Appearance of Attrition

Attrition of the occlusal surfaces is marked by a general flattening of the occlusal or palatal surfaces of the teeth that are engaged during lateral functional movements. The canines are often the most affected teeth. Attrition, unlike erosion, causes wear of amalgam and composite. The amalgam surfaces are often shiny and faceted in the occlusal contact areas. The patient may also have clenching or bruxist habits that may be associated with temporomandibular dysfunction.

With attrition, the worn occlusal and incisal surfaces are flat and come into contact in lateral mandibular movements. A diagnosis of attrition therefore requires that the involved teeth contact in the intercuspal position or in lateral excursion. Erosion tends to accentuate any wear facets (Fig. 5.1), giving the false impression that the patient engages in bruxist activity. Bruxism is often associated with masseteric hypertrophy, temporomandibular joint dysfunction, ridging on the side of the tongue (lingual crenulation) and cervical abfraction lesions on the teeth.

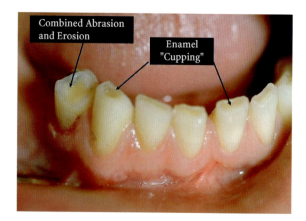

Fig. 5.1 Erosion is a common cause of noncarious tooth tissue loss, often acting in combination with abrasion and attrition

Fig. 5.2 Rapid attrition removes the caries-prone fissure system and early caries

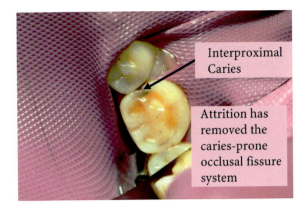

The incidence of occlusal caries in teeth undergoing rapid attrition is low because there is no caries-prone fissure system and early caries is abraded away (Fig. 5.2). In interproximal areas of teeth, caries can initiate and spread unhindered by the occlusal attrition.

5.1.3 Clinical Appearance of Abrasion

Tooth abrasion is often seen as a notching of the cervical surface of the tooth and can be caused by an incorrect toothbrushing technique or using very abrasive toothpastes. Toothbrushes should be made of soft nylon and used with a rotation action, applying only moderate pressure at 45° to the tooth. Gingival recession is often associated with tooth abrasion as it exposes the soft root dentin, which is more easily abraded than enamel.

5.2 Prevention of Toothwear

The general dental practitioner has an important role in advising the patient about their diet, treating symptoms, and monitoring any further tooth loss with study models and photographs. A silicone index of an earlier model can be used to assess rapid toothwear, but often only specific teeth are affected. Only by controlling the etiological factors can further toothwear be reduced, and only when the etiological factors are controlled can treatment be effective. Giving the patient a diet sheet to record their total food consumption over a 3-day period can be a good basis upon which to begin discussion with them. This can be followed by counseling them to avoid erosive foods and drinks. Surface enamel is softened with acidic fluids, but this is increased where the fluid is swirled around the mouth. The patient's oral hygiene habits may be contributing to the tooth substance loss (e.g., an overvigourous scrubbing technique or toothbrushing after acid drinks). Toothbrushing should be avoided for 1 h after consumption of acidic drinks or food, to allow the surface enamel to become remineralized. Sugar-free chewing gum has been shown to stimulate saliva for several hours, and this may have a remineralizing effect on enamel and dentin. Where attrition is the etiological agent, an occlusal splint may be necessary. This can be worn at night.

A treatment plan that satisfies the patient's complaints, is cost-effective, and avoids further tooth reduction is desirable. The vitality of the worn teeth should be checked. Preservation of the remaining teeth and their vitality and the prevention of further toothwear are essential, but the point at which interventive treatment is initiated, if at all, must depend on the patient's particular circumstances. Interventive treatment is not always necessary and can be complicated, especially where teeth lack enough coronal substance to provide retention for restorations. Shortening of the anterior teeth may be a major concern for the patient and initiate their request for urgent treatment, but the toothwear may have been accompanied by dentoalveolar compensation, which maintains the interocclusal space. In these cases, there is reduction of space available for restorations and treatment may therefore be very complicated, requiring surgical crown lengthening, occlusal reorganization, orthodontics, or a Dahl-type appliance (Dahl et al. 1975).

With occlusal reorganization, the study casts are mounted in the retruded contact position (Fig. 5.3a) and not the patient's adopted occlusal position (Fig. 5.3b). The dentist can then visualize the amount of space available for the restorations and produce diagnostic wax-ups. These can be duplicated in stone and a vacuum-formed splint made to assist in construction of the provisional crowns.

With the Dahl concept, the patient has palatal veneer restorations of resin composite bonded to the palatal surface of their anterior teeth. This appliance discludes the posterior teeth, allowing them to erupt, while the anterior teeth are intruded. It can be difficult to accurately mould the composite resin if the palatal additions are made directly in the clinic, and extensive adjustment is usually necessary. An indirect technique is preferred in which the additions to the palatal surface of the anterior teeth are made in wax on a cast, the cast is duplicated, and a vacuum-formed matrix is made. In the clinic the teeth are etched one at a time and bonding agent applied. The resin composite is added to the matrix corresponding to the etched tooth, and light-cured in place. When the additions of resin composite have been made to each of the upper anterior teeth, the centric occlusion is checked and adjusted where necessary

5.2 Prevention of Toothwear

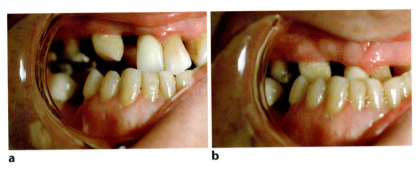

Fig. 5.3 (a) Reorganization of the occlusion can create a space for crowns. This patient has closed into the retruded contact position. (b) The patient has occluded into their habitual closure position or centric occlusion (with maximum intercuspation of their teeth)

so that the posterior teeth are separated by 1–2 mm. Canine guidance is also checked to ensure disclusion of the nonworking side teeth.

Where there has been considerable wear of several teeth, an overdenture may be the preferred treatment option. Advanced treatment requires considerable financial and time commitment from the patient and may require specialist skills from the dentist and technician.

Treatment of Localized Dentinal Sensitivity

One of the commonest complaints from patients is the sudden, sharp sensitivity from eating cold foods, through stimulation of exposed dentin. Dentinal sensitivity results from the movement of fluid in the tubules, causing stimulation of pulpal nerve endings. Blocking these tubules should therefore stop the pain. The anesthetized tooth should be cleaned with pumice, washed, and the affected area blot dried. A desensitizing agent such as Gluma Desensitizer (Heraeus Kultzer) is applied for 30 s and then the area dried. This desenstizing agent will stop dentinal fluid flow. Gluma Desensitizer contains 5% glutaraldehyde and 35% HEMA, and therefore contact with the patient's soft tissues should be avoided. The glutaraldehyde has a strong antibacterial action, but its main method of action is occlusion of the dentinal fluid by precipitation of serum proteins within it. There are other desensitizing products available, but some may affect the bond strength of subsequently applied resin composite. Gluma Desensitizer is compatible with any restorative material and does not affect the bonding of subsequently applied adhesive agents. It cannot be used to treat the pain from irreversible pulpitis.

5.3
Recent Developments in the Treatment of Tooth Wear

Adhesively retained ceramic and composite restorations offer the possibility of conservative restoration of teeth without causing iatrogenic damage in already worn teeth. Provided the restoration has enough enamel for satisfactory adhesion, adhesive dentistry allows the retention of restorations in severely worn teeth. By avoiding conventional crown preparations, the vitality of teeth in the young patient is more likely to be preserved. In addition, crown lengthening followed by conventional crowns has the disadvantage that the crowns often look triangular and misshapen.

5.3.1
Noncarious Cervical Restorations

Amalgam has been largely replaced by composite resin, resin-modified glass ionomer, and glass ionomer restorations in the treatment of cervical lesions. This is because these materials have good esthetics and mechanical properties and are capable of being bonded to enamel and dentin. Microfill resin composites usually have better esthetics than the glass ionomer materials and an improved resistance to an acid environment. They can be highly polished and resist abrasion very well. Failure of cervical restorations may be primarily due to flexure of the tooth, rupturing the bond between the tooth and the restorative material. Microfill resin composites tend to be less stiff and therefore flex with the tooth in function. A successful bond of resin composite to the dentin in the cervical region can be difficult as the dentin is often sclerotic and provides an unfavorable bond surface. Acid-eroded dentin is often sclerotic. Beveling the enamel margin improves the retention of resin composite and resin-modified glass ionomer materials (such as GC Fuji II LC Improved, manufactured by GC America, IL, USA; Uno et al. 1997). Beveling the gingival margins located on dentin or cementum is not recommended, as this has been shown to increase the microleakage in restorations restored with resin composite or compomer (Owens et al. 1998).

5.3.2
Clinical Procedures for Restoration of Cervical Lesions

Fuji II LC (GC America) is a resin-modified glass ionomer restorative that is suitable for restoring class V cavities. The powder is an aluminosilicate powder and the liquid contains polyacrylic acid, tartaric acid, camphorquinone, and various resins such as HEMA. The material has good radiopacity and releases fluoride, although whether the fluoride release results in a significant clinical caries-inhibitive effect is not known. After completion of the cavity preparation, a GC Cavity Conditioner (containing 20% polyacrylic acid and 3% aluminum chloride) is applied to the moist dentin for 10 s to remove the smear layer. It has been shown recently that if the smear layer is allowed to remain, it may hydrolyze over time, allowing bacterial penetration and microleakage. The capsules are activated by pushing the plunger and triturating them for 10 s. Once the cement is mixed it is applied to the moist cavity. The incorporation of air bubbles must be avoided. The material is contoured with a plastic matrix strip and light-cured for 20 s, which will polymerize the material to a depth of 2 mm. If the cavity depth is greater than this, a layering technique must be used. Excess material is removed by polishing with a superfine diamond bur and polishing strips and discs. GC Fuji Varnish is applied to seal the restoration if the material has been exposed to the air during polymerization.

Dyract AP is a compomer material that is used in conjunction with Prime and Bond NTtm adhesive. The manufacturer states that it is not necessary to etch the cavity preparation in non-stress-bearing class V restorations, but where no tooth preparation has taken place the cavity preparation should be cleaned with a rubber cup and a pumice slurry. The Prime and Bond NTtm adhesive is applied generously to the cavity to cover the enamel and dentin and then gently dried for 5 s to evaporate the solvent. This adhesive combines a primer and adhesive resin in one container. The surface should appear glossy, and if not then further applications of adhesive are required. The adhesive is light-cured for 10 s and the Dyract AP restorative applied and light-cured for 40 s.

5.3.3
Why Do Cervical Restorations Fail?

Masticatory forces cause cuspal flexure and the stresses are concentrated in the cervical lesion, tending to dislodge restorative materials in this region. Resin-modified glass ionomers are about twice as flexible as glass ionomers and are therefore more likely to be retained during flexing of the tooth. In addition, they absorb water for several days after photostabilization and the resulting expansion tends to offset the shrinkage caused by the initial set of the resin components. If resin composite alone is used to restore cervical lesions, poor marginal adaptation at the gingival margin is inevitable (Gordon et al. 1991). This is mainly caused by polymerization shrinkage away from the gingival surface due to poor adhesion at the dentin surface. Another reason for the poor marginal adaptation of resin composites may be the difference in the coefficient of linear thermal expansion between restorative material and tooth. The coefficient of linear thermal expansion for dentin is about $11 \times 10^{-6}/^{\circ}C$ (Xu et al. 1989), whereas the coefficient is $33 \times 10^{-6}/^{\circ}C$ (Sideridou et al. 2004) for a typical "universal" resin composite suitable for anterior and posterior tooth restoration, such as Filtek Z250 (3M ESPE, MN, USA). The major factor affecting the coefficient of thermal expansion of resin composites is the filler content, and highly filled composites are recommended to prevent microleakage resulting from the effects of temperature fluctuations in the mouth.

Subgingival, cervical resin-composite restorations are easily contaminated by gingival exudate (Fig. 5.4a). The application of a retraction cord soaked with a drop of astringent solution to the gingival sulcus can prevent subsequent contamination of the restoration with blood and gingival fluid. The gingival tissues retract after a few minutes and allow the margin of the restoration to be finished more easily without further gingival trauma (Fig. 5.4b).

"Sandwich" restorations of glass ionomer and resin composite have been used as a way of reducing the polymerization shrinkage by reducing the amount of resin composite and minimizing the adverse effects of microleakage. Glass ionomers release fluoride, which should theoretically reduce the incidence of secondary caries. A thin layer of glass ionomer is applied to the base of the cervical cavity and primer/adhesive resin applied to the beveled, etched enamel and dentinal walls. Resin composite is added to the cavity, contoured, and polymerized.

Glass ionomer restorations fail primarily as a result of marginal fracture. This material is often used in the class V situation where the material is subjected to flexural stress. The brittleness of glass ionomer may contribute

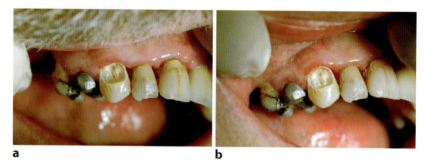

Fig. 5.4 (a) During placement of the resin composite for this deep subgingival restoration, contamination by gingival exudates is possible. (b) Placement of retraction cord and astringent solution for 2 min allowed the gingival tissues to retract

to fracture in this stress-bearing location. However, because glass ionomer materials release fluoride, dentists may choose these materials in patients with poor oral hygiene to utilize the anticariogenic properties of this material. It may therefore be poor patient oral hygiene as well as the inherent brittleness of glass ionomer that causes the mean restoration longevity to be only a few years in some studies (Burke et al. 1999).

5.3.4
New Developments in Direct Posterior Resin Composites

Using modern adhesive systems, tooth removal is primarily limited to removing caries. Overhanging enamel margins are retained as they will be strengthened by adhesive bonding. Manufacturers are investing considerable effort in developing simplified adhesive and resin-composite restorative systems with the minimum of office steps and the widest range of applications. An example of a single-step adhesive is iBond (Heraeus Kultzer, NY, USA). Three consecutive layers of iBond are applied generously to the clean, dry cavity. The adhesive is gently massaged for 30 s, dried gently with air, and then polymerized for 20 s. Venus (Heraeus Kultzer) is applied to the cavity using an incremental technique and each addition is polymerized for 20 s. Venus is a typical hybrid resin-composite material with submicron barium glass filler particles (average particle size of 0.7 µm) and is suitable for onlay and inlay applications, as well as direct composite veneers.

Another single-step, self-etching dental adhesive, Xeno III (manufactured by Dentsply Caulk, DE, USA), contains a fluoride-releasing, polyfunctional methacrylate resin and phosphoric-acid-modified methacrylate. Equal amounts of the two components are mixed for 5 s and applied generously to the class V cavity. The adhesive material is left for 20 s, dried gently, and then light-cured for at least 10 s. A low-shrinkage composite material (such as Quixx, manufactured by Dentsply Caulk) is then applied and light-cured. Quixx is a posterior restorative designed for class I and II cavity restoration. The material is finished using finishing diamonds and polishing discs (e.g., Soflex discs; 3M Dental Products, St. Paul, MN, USA). One Gloss is a system of alumina- and silica-impregnated synthetic rubber points (manufactured by Shofu Dental Corporation, CA, USA) designed to polish composite resin (Fig. 5.5). The points are used with a feather-light touch (0.3 N) and at a recommended speed of 3,000–10,000 rpm. Final polishing can be obtained with SuperBuff (Shofu Dental Corporation), which is an abrasive-impregnated disc that avoids the use of polishing paste. This system requires that the surface is wet prior to polishing and a light pressure is used during polishing.

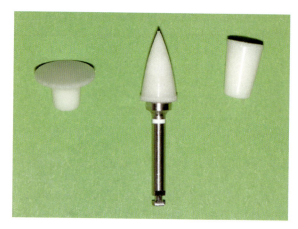

Fig. 5.5 Alumina- and silica-impregnated synthetic rubber points designed for polishing the resin composite

5.3.5
Addition of Resin Composite to Anterior Teeth

Spacing between the teeth can result from erosion, and the patient may request closure of the spaces between the teeth. In many cases the teeth are also reduced in height so that restoring only the width will result in an unsatisfactory result (Fig. 5.6a). Impressions should be taken and the cast modified with wax so that the patient can visualize the result prior to restorative treatment. A clear acrylic splint constructed from the modified casts can be helpful in copying the agreed shape of the teeth in the wax-up. However, using the splint as a matrix for the resin composite can result in the composite additions bond-

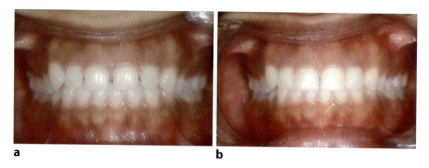

Fig. 5.6 (a) Long-term consumption of carbonated beverages had caused mild erosive wear of the upper teeth with spacing and thinning of the enamel. (b) Closure of the spaces between the upper incisor teeth was made with resin composite additions

ing to each other. Greater control can be achieved by hand-carving the resin composite prior to curing (Fig. 5.6b) or else using the plint with alternate teeth.

Some patients request closure of diastemas formed as a result of erosion of their anterior teeth. Because the labial enamel of the anterior teeth has been reduced in thickness by the erosive processes, tooth reduction is rarely necessary to create enough space for layering of different shades of resin composite. The labial surface of the maxillary incisors lies in three planes with the curved gingival third, leading to a relatively flat middle region and a palatally inclined incisal edge. Minimizing the labial surface lobes and depressions of the resin composite restoration, as well as a minimal incisal embrasure gives an appearance of a wider tooth.

Planning the position of the incisal edge of the restoration is necessary to avoid traumatic interference of the resin composite in protrusion and lateral excursive movements. The position of the facioproximal line angles can alter the apparent width of the teeth; closely approximated line angles give a narrow tooth appearance.

Gradia Direct is a light-cured microfilled hybrid resin composite. Clinically, UniFil Bond Self-Etching Primer is applied to the interproximal surfaces. The enamel of the adjacent tooth is protected with a matrix strip. After 20 s, the tooth is gently dried. UniFil Bond is then applied to the primed enamel surface, and light-cured for 20 s. Gradia Direct resin composite is then applied to the surface and cured for 20 s.

5.3.6
Developments in Indirect Resin Composite Technology

In extensive posterior cavities, providing direct composite restorations with the correct tooth shape and tight interproximal contact can be a formidable task. Indirect resin composites avoid these disadvantages because they are prepared on a laboratory die rather than the tooth itself, and polymerization shrinkage is limited to the luting resin cement. The interfacial gap between the restoration and the tooth is therefore much reduced with indirect restorations (Iida et al. 2003). When two materials with different stiffnesses are joined together and a force is applied, stresses are always concentrated at the interface. The elastic modulus of many composites is therefore somewhat similar to that of dentin, although there is evidence from finite-element analysis studies that indirect resin composites and luting cements with a low elastic modulus dissipate applied loads because of their ability to deform (Ausiello et al. 2004). The stress applied to the remaining tooth is therefore less.

Resins also avoid any wear of opposing teeth, which is a complication associated with roughened porcelain surfaces. After adjusting porcelain it is possible to polish the surface, but this is time consuming. Indirect resin-composite restorations are easier to adjust.

5.3.6.1
Targis/Vectris Crowns

The Targis restorative system combines the Targis Ceromer (Ceramic Optimized Polymer, Ivoclar) restorative material with a Vectris fiber-reinforced composite (Vivadent). The teeth are prepared for single anterior or posterior crowns with a 1.5- to 2.0-mm reduction on the occlusal surfaces, 1.5-mm reduction on the axial walls, and 1.0-mm reduction at the supragingival margin. All internal line angles should be rounded. The axial walls must have no undercut. The material is bonded to the tooth using an adhesive dual cure resin (Ivoclar Cem Kit Variolink II).

5.3.6.2
Sinfony

This indirect microhybrid composite material (3M-ESPE) is suitable for inlays/onlays, veneers, and full crowns. The preparation guidelines for crowns are identical to those of Targis/Vectris. Preparation guidelines for molar inlays or onlays must allow a minimum thickness of 1.5mm of material to allow sufficient strength to the restoration. The cavosurface margin must be a butt joint. All internal line angles are rounded.

Sinfony contains aliphatic and cycloaliphatic monomers and aluminum glass (50wt%) and silica fillers (Kakaboura et al. 2003). It has a wide range of enamel, dentin, opaque, and transparent shades. In the laboratory, Sinfony is applied to the cavity restoration and photopolymerized for 15s. It then undergoes a secondary photopolymerization cure under vacuum for 15min in 3M ESPE's Visio-Beta machine. Sinfony has been recently shown to have improved fracture resistance when combined with fiber reinforcement (Lehmann et al. 2004).

Sinfony indirect laboratory composite can be bonded to metal copings using a chemical adhesive system (Rocatec bonding system, 3M-ESPE). In this procedure, a silane layer is applied to the sandblasted coping. Opaque, dentin and enamel composite layers are then applied and polymerized to obtain the final crown shape.

5.3.6.3
Belleglass HP

This indirect resin composite (SDS-Kerr) contains aliphatic urethane monomers, and has a high inorganic filler content. It is polymerized in two stages;

firstly under photopolymerization for 40 s and then the secondary polymerization is carried out in the nitrogen atmosphere of a Belleglass curing unit at 140 °C and 60 psi pressure (where 1 psi = 6.89 kPa) for 20 min. The cured material has a high degree of conversion.

5.3.6.4
Other Fiber Systems

Other fiber systems are on the market whereby the dentist or technician must incorporate the resin composite into the fiber network. These indirect-composite restorations are cemented on the etched tooth with a dual-cure adhesive resin cement.

5.4
Ceramic Inlay and Onlay Restorations

These ceramic restorations are adhesively retained with a resin cement, while the tooth surface must be treated with a conditioner and dentin bonding agent. Because ceramic materials can be etched to form a roughened surface, the adhesive bond of porcelain restorations is more reliable than that achieved with indirect resin composites. They are increasingly in demand from patients requesting a more esthetic option, but they are more time consuming and technically demanding, and are therefore more expensive than the traditional restorative techniques using gold. Indirect porcelain restorative materials have excellent mechanical properties, tissue biocompatibility, color stability, and abrasion resistance.

Kelly and Smales (2004) have shown that the traditional cast gold onlay is one of the least cost-effective, indirect posterior restorative options, and indirect porcelain onlays are likely to prove to be no more cost-effective. When dentists are undergoing treatment themselves, most still prefer traditional gold and amalgam restorations rather than the esthetic alternatives (Rosenstiel et al. 2004). In trying to assess the longevity of ceramic restorations, most studies have been short term and performed in a university setting where time pressures on the operator are less. Some concern has been expressed about the progressive wear of the composite luting agent giving rise to marginal discoloration and secondary caries. A highly filled, viscous luting cement is recommended because it is associated with lower polymerization stress and microleakage (Hahn et al. 2001). Bulk fracture of some of the ceramic materials due to the inherent brittleness of the material has also been observed, but this may be due to incorrect tooth preparation. In a study by Molin and Karlsson (2000), 8% of the ceramic inlays (Cerec, Mirage, and Empress) were bulk fractured over a follow-up period of 5 years. Posterior occlusal onlays are an esthetic adhesive restoration, but debonding and fracture is reported as common, especially when retention can only be obtained from dentin and the restoration is subjected to bruxist grinding (Walls et al. 2002). Over an approximately 5-year observation period, there was 9.7% failure of extensive dentin/enamel bonded posterior ceramic restorations in nonvital teeth in a study by van Dijken et al. (2001), but only a 6.6% failure in vital teeth. The majority of the restorations failed as a result of fracture, emphasizing the need for sufficient bulk of ceramic material.

Patients often request the replacement of amalgam restorations with resin-bonded porcelain inlays and onlays, which are a more esthetic replacement for amalgam. Unfortunately, the undercuts on the teeth are frequently removed at the expense of further widening of the occlusal isthmus. Blocking out undercuts with glass ionomer cements should be considered. Etemadi et al. (1999) examined 57 tooth preparations for posterior resin-bonded porcelain onlays and found that the occlusal isthmus widths were approximately two-thirds of the intercuspal widths, and wider than expected. However, luted indirect restorations restore the tooth to its original intact strength (Dalpino et al. 2002).

5.5
Inlay Restorations

Finite-element analysis has been used to derive some of the principles of preparation of posterior resin-bonded inlay restorations. Evidence would indicate that the gingival floors of the cavity should be flat with 90° cavosurface

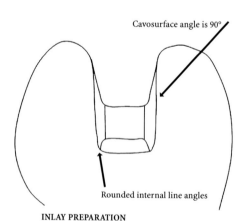

Fig. 5.7 Inlay preparation

angles, finishing in enamel wherever possible (Fig. 5.7). Internal line angles should be rounded. Bevelling of the margins creates weak porcelain margins and should be avoided. Each axial surface should diverge from the vertical by about 10°. Undercuts can be blocked out with a glass ionomer cement. A eugenol-free temporary cement must be used to cement the provisional restoration. Eugenol may prevent the polymerization of the resin-composite cement.

Feldspathic Porcelain Inlays and Onlays

These restorations are fired on phosphate-bonded working models and then re-fitted to the master model (Fig. 5.8a). The original die is duplicated in the refractory material. The porcelain is applied to the hardened refractory surface and fired. The final esthetic result is usually satisfactory (Fig. 5.8b), but concerns have been expressed about whether these inlays are strong enough to resist masticatory forces. In the case illustrated in Fig. 5.8, the lateral forces on the premolar onlay were protected by a canine-guided occlusion.

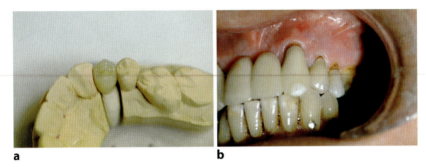

Fig. 5.8 (a) Feldspathic porcelain inlays and onlays are fired on phosphate-bonded working models and then refitted to the master model. (b) Feldspathic porcelain onlay restoring the upper premolar. These restorations have excellent esthetics, but fracture easily

5.6 Onlay Restorations

Sufficient resistance to occlusal forces can only be provided by at least 1.5 – 2 mm of occlusal reduction to allow a sufficient thickness of porcelain (Fig. 5.9). Internal line angles should be rounded. Beveled margins are contraindicated as they provide thin porcelain margins that are easily fractured, but instead the cavosurfaces should finish with a 90° butt-joint or chamfer margins (Fig. 5.10). In a finite-element study, Abu-Hassan et al. (2000) showed that a sufficient thickness of porcelain was necessary at the buccal margin of the restoration to resist horizontal loads, which arise during mastication and are potentially more damaging than vertical loads. Each axial surface should taper about 10° from the vertical, which is slightly greater than that generally recommended for conventional cast gold inlays. The increased taper allows a greater thickness of porcelain and increased strength, and because the porcelain is bonded to the tooth with a dentin bonding agent and dual-cured resin cement, there is little loss of retention. The increased internal taper of these restorations will tend to increase the occlusal isthmus width, but this will reduce the stress on the remaining tooth structure (Manhart et al. 1996). Retentive grooves are not indicated.

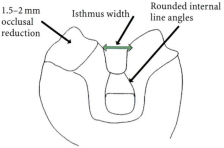

Fig. 5.9 Resin-bonded porcelain onlay

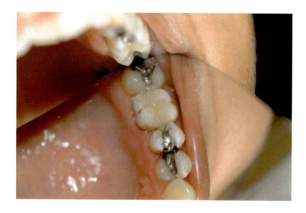

Fig. 5.10 All inlay and onlay porcelain restorations require a 90° cavosurface butt joint

5.6.1
Milled Ceramic Inlays or Onlays

5.6.1.1
Cerec 3

Using Cerec 3 (Sirona, Dental Systems GmbH, Bensheim, Germany), titanium dioxide powder is placed on the preparation, an optical impression taken and the restoration is designed on the computer screen. When the dentist is satisfied with his design it is forwarded to the milling machine, which prepares the restoration in ceramic. This can then be cemented at the same appointment. The technique is suitable for veneers, crowns, and onlays as well as inlays. A summary of the success rate of Cerec inlays and onlays is given in Table 5.1.

Table 5.1 Summary of the success rate of Cerec inlays and onlays

Cerec Inlay Success Rates	
Sjögren et al. (2004)	89% Survival after 10 years
Posselt and Kerschbaum (2003)	95.5% Survival after 9 years
Reiss (1994)	91.9% survival after 6 years
Martin and Jedynakiewicz (1999)	97.4% over a period of 4.2 years
Cerec Inlay and Onlay Success Rate	
Otto and De Nisco (2002)	90.4% success after 10 years

There has been insufficient research to establish what constitutes an acceptable width of marginal gap under an indirect restoration. Marginal gaps of Cerec 3 crown restorations in independent studies have been reported as ranging from 53 to 67 µm, which is excellent (Nakamura et al. 2003). Other studies have found that inlays milled using the CEREC 3 system were more accurately fitting than those milled using the CEREC 2 system, although marginal gaps for both were less than 50 µm (Estefan et al. 2003). The use of high-viscosity luting agents may increase the marginal gaps, but these materials have better wear resistance. The luted restoration is polished using Soflex discs grit sizes 150, 360, 600, and 1,200 (3M, USA). Cerec crowns have a higher mean fracture load than that reported for the average maximum masticatory force, with no significant difference in the mean fracture resistance of the unprepared natural teeth and that of computer-aided design and computer aided manufacture (CAD/CAM)-produced all-ceramic bonded crowns (Attia and Kern 2004). A study of more than 1,000 Cerec inlays revealed a failure rate after 6 years of 9.1% (Reiss 1994).

Each surface is capable of detailed modification. The interproximal surface can be designed precisely. The occlusal surface can be modified using an optical impression of a centric occlusion registration, or the original occlusal surface prior to preparation can be copied. Elastomeric impressions, provisional restorations, and the services of a laboratory technician are not required for this technique. The effect of adhesive bonding in Cerec 3 may be more important than the strength of the ceramic materials used, as stronger materials such as In-Ceram Spinell have a similar clinical success rate. In a dental-office-based study, 2,328 ceramic inlays were placed in 794 patients (Posselt and Kerschbaum 2003). The restorations were manufactured at the chairside using Cerec technology and adhesively inserted at the same appointment. The probability of survival of the restorations was 95.5% after 9 years, which is excellent. Similar excellent survival figures have been reported by Sjögren et al. (2004), who found that 89% of the 61 Cerec inlays functioned well after 10 years. Most failures occur as a result of ceramic or tooth fracture.

5.6.1.2
IPS Empress System

This pressable glass ceramic technique (Ivoclar Vivadent, Schaan, Liechtenstein) utilizes feldspathic porcelain reinforced with 35%vol of leucite. It is suitable for fabrication of inlays, onlays, crowns, and veneers, and has a flexural strength of up to 120 MPa. The inlay is waxed-up and invested. The ceramic ingot is heated to 1,200 °C and the softened material pressed into the mould. Following disinvestment, the inlay can be glazed with pigment shades. For anterior crowns or veneers, the restoration is cut back and leucite-reinforced ceramics can be added by conventional sintering. Etching the internal surface of the IPS Empress inlay with 10% hydrofluoric acid, followed by silane treatment, has been shown to be more effective than sandblasting with alumina followed by silane (Spohr et al. 2003). The IPS Empress restorations are etched for 60 s using IPS Ceramic Etching Gel (Ivoclar Vivadent), washed, dried, and then adhesively cemented. Bonding procedures should be carried out under a rubber dam to prevent salivary contamination. Excess luting agent should be removed. In an interesting study, Hekland et al. (2003) showed that most remakes and problems associated with all-ceramic inlays/onlays, veneers, and crowns occur before rather than after cementation. Once cemented, these restorations have an excellent survival.

Empress II is a glass ceramic composed of lithium disilicate and lithium orthophosphate. This material has improved strength over the leucite-reinforced materials, and has excellent esthetics due to its high translucency. The Empress II restoration is manufactured by a hot-press process at 920 °C, using the lost wax method. The esthetic surface layer is provided by a layering ceramic composed of apatite glass. The flexural strength is very high (about 400 MPa) because the crystals deflect the propogation of cracks through the material. The appearance of the patient illustrated in Fig. 5.11a was improved immensely by providing Empress II crowns on 12, 11, and 21 (Fig. 5.11b,c). At a later date, the upper left lateral incisor tooth was re-crowned and a Procera crown was constructed (Fig. 5.11d). The crown was luted in place using a glass ionomer luting agent (Fig. 5.11e) and the excess cement removed. The patient was delighted with the aesthetic result (Fig. 5.11f).

Studies have shown that IPS Empress inlays and onlays have a good survival rate (96% at 4.5 years, declining to 91% at 7 years; Brochu and El-Mowafy 2002; Chadwick 2004). Bulk fracture is the main reason for failure, indicating that restorations require sufficient reduction to allow enough ceramic to be used, especially in the isthmus region.

In view of the reported bulk fracture of porcelain inlay restorations in some studies due to occlusal trauma, hyperocclusion must be avoided. The occlusion can only be adjusted when the onlay/inlay restorations have been luted in position. The occlusion is adjusted with fine diamonds and polishing paste. The strength of a ceramic is governed by the surface roughness of the restoration (de Jager et al. 2000). It can be very time consuming and difficult to polish the occlusal surface of porcelain restorations. It may be the residual roughness in the porcelain restoration that predisposes it to microcracking and bulk failure of the material. Although direct and indirect porcelain restorations have a good survival rate, failure of these restorations is due to secondary caries or bulk fracture (Thordrup et al. 2001).

5.6.1.3
Fortress

This is another leucite-reinforced porcelain used for the fabrication of anterior and posterior crowns, inlays/onlays, and veneers (Chameleon Dental, KS, USA). It has a flexural strength of 175–180 MPa, but derives most of its strength from the adhesive bond to the tooth. A thick ceramic powder and water slurry is applied to a refractory die and sintered, and the restoration is built up in layers.

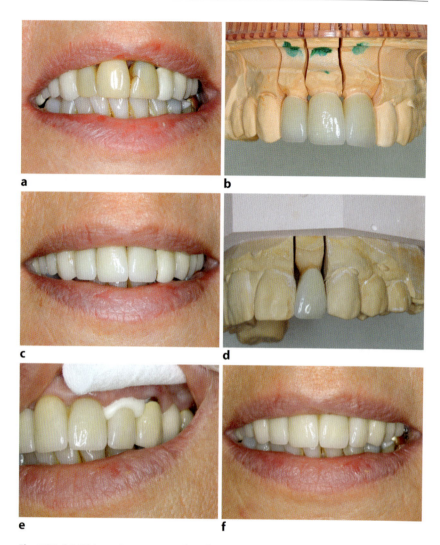

Fig. 5.11 (a) This patient presented with an unsightly color mismatch of previously constructed crowns and natural teeth. (b) Empress II crowns were constructed on 12, 11, and 21. (c) The Empress II crowns after cementation. (d) At a later date, the upper left lateral incisor tooth was recrowned and a Procera crown was constructed. (e) The Procera crown on the upper left lateral incisor tooth was luted in place using a glass ionomer luting agent. (f) The esthetic results with Procera and Empress II are excellent

5.7
Full-Veneer Posterior Porcelain Crowns

A list of the ceramics available for posterior restorative applications is given in Table 5.2. Because optimal esthetics and an excellent gingival response are observed with ceramic materials, techniques such as resin-bonded all-ceramic crowns are often indicated in patients with toothwear. However, these patients have already lost considerable amounts of tooth tissue, so further tooth reduction by the dentist must be judged in the individual patient. Guidelines suggest that posterior full-veneer coverage requires an axial reduction of 1–1.5 mm, and an occlusal reduction of 1.5–2 mm, with a heavy chamfer or butt margin (of angle 90–120°). Ceramic crowns must not be cemented using resin-modified glass ionomers as these materials undergo a postset expansion that can split the restoration.

Table 5.2 Ceramics available for posterior restorative applications

Veneers	Inlays or Onlays	Full veneer crown
Empress system	Empress system	*Procera AllCeram
Cerec system	Cerec system	*In-Ceram
		Empress system
		Cerec system
		Lava

* In-Ceram and *Procera cannot be effectively etched because they have a low silica content. The fit surface must be sandblasted with 50-μm Al_2O_3 particles using an air pressure of 2.5 bar and ultrasonically cleaned in 96% isopropyl alcohol, and silane added. The restorations can be luted using a dual-cured composite resin luting agent

5.7.1
In-Ceram

Glass-infiltrated In-Ceram ceramic cores were developed in the 1980s. In-Ceram Spinell (a mixture of magnesia and alumina) has good translucency and can be used for single anterior crowns, while In-Ceram Alumina and In-Ceram Zirconia are recommended for single posterior crowns. In-Ceram materials (developed by Vita Zahnfabrik, Bad Säckingen, Germany) have excellent strength (Sobrinho et al. 1998) because the spinel ($MgAl_2O_4$), alumina, or zirconia core acts to prevent crack propagation from the fitting surface through the ceramic. When veneered with a 10% aluminum oxide content

Vitadur Alpha porcelain (Viadent, Bria, CA, USA) the esthetic results are excellent. Unlike the pressable ceramics, In-Ceram materials are not dependent on a resin bond to the tooth to provide strength to the restoration.

VITA In-Ceram Alumina and Zirconia blocks are available in presintered blocks that are easily milled using Cerec technology (Sirona, Dental Systems) to produce a coping crown substructure. This presintered coping is then infiltrated with glass at 1,100 °C and the crown formed in traditional porcelain. The fitting surface of the In-Ceram crown is sand-blasted with 50-µm-diameter aluminum oxide at 80 psi (Ad Abrader; J. Morita USA, Irvine, CA, USA) for 3 s. The restoration is cleaned then luted with an adhesive resin cement. Super-Bond C&B (manufactured by Sun Medical, Shiga, Japan) is a resin cement that contains 4-META, and which has performed particularly well as an adhesive luting agent in in vitro tests (Komine et al. 2004). It is a ductile cement with a low modulus of elasticity and high fracture toughness, which provides a stress-distributing function during loading of the In-Ceram crown.

A 94% success over 3 years has been reported for In-Ceram posterior crowns (McClaren and White 2000) compared with a 95.35% success over a similar mean period of 37 months with IPS Empress crowns (Fradeani and Aquilano 1997).

5.7.2
Procera AllCeram Crowns

Procera AllCeram crowns (developed by Nobel Biocare, Gotenburg, Sweden) have an alumina core designed from a digital scan of the master die. The core is very dense, with a high flexural strength, and is made by sintering alumina at 1,600–1,700 °C from a digital prescription. Procera AllCeram can be used in inlays, onlays, and crowns in the anterior or posterior region of the mouth (Andersson et al. 1998).

The tooth preparation should have rounded internal line angles, so boxes and grooves are contraindicated. There is a reduction of 2.0 mm on the occlusal surface and 1.5 mm on the axial wall. After the die is trimmed, it is scanned and the data fed into a computer program, which designs a coping (0.4–0.6 mm in thickness). To facilitate the digitization process, a chamfered margin is required. As with other porcelain and indirect-composite systems, the preparation must be rounded with an absence of sharp margins or undercut. The coping design incorporates a 20% enlargement, which compensates for the shrinkage of the alumina during sintering. The design information is transmitted to a production station (Fair Law, New Jersey, USA) where the alumina coping is constructed. Compatible feldspathic porcelain (AllCeram Porcelain, Ducera) are added to the core to produce excellent esthetics.

5.8 Cementation of the Restoration

It is recommended that Procera AllCeram crowns are cemented with a chemically cured resin cement (such as Panavia 21; Kuraray, Japan; Albert et al. 2004) or dual-cure resin, as these provide the least microleakage. Glass ionomer is recommended as the luting agent when moisture control is difficult.

Studies have shown that Procera AllCeram has an excellent precision of fit, with gaps of less than 70 µm (May et al. 1998). Oden et al. (1998) evaluated the clinical performance of 100 Procera AllCeram crowns after 5 years. Of the 97 restorations available, 5 had experienced fractures and 1 recurrent caries. The remaining restorations were ranked as excellent or satisfactory in terms of color, shape, and marginal integrity. The Procera AllCeram technique is expensive though, requiring special laboratory scanning equipment and technician training. Fig. 5.12 illustrates upper anterior Procera crowns that are now 8 years old and functioning very satisfactorily.

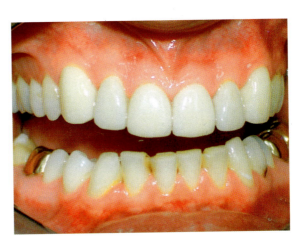

Fig. 5.12 Upper anterior Procera crowns that are now 8 years old and functioning very satisfactorily. Placement of well-fitting crown margins at the gingival margin produced an excellent gingival response

5.8
Cementation of the Restoration

Application of retraction cord to the gingival sulcus prior to cementation can prevent moisture contamination during cementation. In addition, the retraction cord prevents the gingival tissues from interfering with the seating of the restoration and allows easy visualization of excess cement. Excess cement can be removed with a scalpel.

5.9
Choosing the Correct Restorative System

New developments in ceramic and composite systems have increased the choice of restoratives available for the dentist in treating noncarious tooth loss. It has often been stated that patients requiring a crown, but who have a history of bruxism, are best treated using the traditional metal-ceramic crown because only this restoration has sufficient strength. However, the most recent crown and bridge ceramic systems have outstanding strength. The latest addition to the all-ceramic family is a polycrystalline, zirconia-based Lava ceramic (3M ESPE), which has exceptional strength and can be used for anterior and posterior crowns and bridges. Anterior crown preparations are similar to those required for porcelain fused to metal restorations, and require a 1.0- to 1.5-mm labial and lingual reduction and a 1.5- to 2.0-mm incisal reduction. Posterior crown preparations require a 1- to 2-mm axial reduction and a 1.5- to 2.0-mm occlusal clearance. A chamfer margin and rounded internal preparation contours should be produced. Lava restorations have an excellent marginal fit because they are constructed using CAD/CAM from presintered zirconia blanks. Traditional cements are used to lute the Lava restoration, which simplifies luting procedures. Because of the high strength of Lava restorations, tooth preparation can be less severe than using other glass-infiltrated ceramic materials.

Figure 5.13a illustrates a patient who requested an esthetic improvement to their upper incisors. The upper right central had to be extracted and was eventually replaced with a fixed partial denture using Lava technology

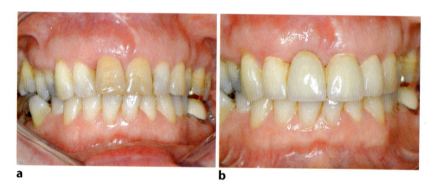

Fig. 5.13 (a) This patient requested an esthetic improvement to their dark yellowish-brown upper incisors. (b) The upper right central was extracted and replaced with a fixed partial denture using Lava technology. In addition, the upper left lateral incisor received a Lavacrown. There was an excellent esthetic improvement

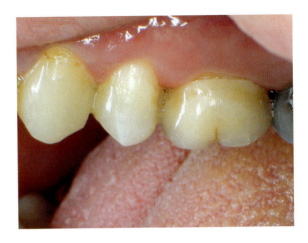

Fig. 5.14 Lava technology was used in replacing the upper first molar, producing a restoration with excellent esthetics and strength

(Fig. 5.13b). In addition, the upper left lateral incisor received a Lava crown. Figure 5.14 illustrates the use of Lava technology in replacing an upper first molar, producing a restoration with excellent esthetics and strength.

5.10 Conclusion

Noncarious tooth tissue loss provides a challenge of diagnosis and treatment for the dental surgeon. For example, some patients find it difficult to discuss their eating disorder problems, often denying that their diet or vomiting can be affecting their teeth. Oral health-care providers have a crucial role in the early identification of eating disorders and in the referral and management of these patients. Adhesive technology can be used to treat toothwear and should simplify treatment for this increasingly common problem, producing restorations with excellent appearance and functionality.

References

Abu-Hassan MI, Abu-Hammad OA, Harrison A. Stress distribution associated with loaded ceramic onlay restorations with different designs of marginal preparation. An FEA study. J Oral Rehabil 2000; 27:294–298.

Albert FE, El-Mowafy OM. Marginal adaptation and microleakage of Procera AllCeram crowns with four cements. Int J Prosthodont 2004; 17:529–35.

Andersson M, Razzoog ME, Oden A, Hegenbarth EA, Lang BR. Procera: a new way to achieve an all-ceramic crown. Quintessence Int 1998; 29:285–296.

Attia A, Kern M. Fracture strength of all-ceramic crowns luted using two bonding methods. J Prosthet Dent 2004; 91:247–252.

Ausiello P, Rengo S, Davidson CL, Watts DC. Stress distributions in adhesively cemented ceramic and resin-composite Class II inlay restorations: a 3D-FEA study. Dent Mater 2004; 20:862–872.

Brochu JF, El-Mowafy O. Longevity and clinical performance of IPS-Empress ceramic restorations – a literature review. J Can Dent Assoc 2002; 68:233–237.

Burke FJT, Cheung SW, Mjor IA, Wilson NHF. Restoration longevity and analysis of reasons for the placement and replacement of restorations provided by vocational dental practitioners and their trainers in the United Kingdom. Quintessence Int 1999; 30:234–242.

Chadwick B. Good short-term survival of IPS-Empress crowns. Evid Based Dent 2004; 5:73.

Dahl BL, Krogstad O, Karlsen K. An alternative treatment in cases with advanced localized attrition. J Oral Rehabil 1975; 2:209–214.

Dalpino PH, Francischone CE, Ishikiriama A, Franco EB. Fracture resistance of teeth directly and indirectly restored with composite resin and indirectly restored with ceramic materials. Am J Dent 2002; 15:389–394.

De Jager N, Feilzer AJ, Davidson CL. The influence of surface roughness on porcelain strength. Dent Mater 2000; 16:381–388.

Estafan D, Dussetschleger F, Agosta C, Reich S. Scanning electron microscope evaluation of CEREC II and CEREC III inlays. Gen Dent 2003; 51:450–454.

Etemadi S, Smales RJ, Drummond PW, Goodhart JR. Assessment of tooth preparation designs for posterior resin-bonded porcelain restorations. J Oral Rehabil 1999; 26:691–697.

Fradeani M, Aquilano A. Clinical experience with Empress crowns. Int J Prosthodont 1997 10:241–247.

Gordon M, Wasserstein A, Gorfil C, Imber S. Microleakage in three designs of glass ionomer under composite resin restorations. J Oral Rehabil 1991; 18:149–154.

Hahn P, Attin T, Grofke M, Hellwig E. Influence of resin cement viscosity on microleakage of ceramic inlays. Dent Mater 2001; 17:191–196.

Hekland H, Riise T, Berg E. Remakes of Colorlogic and IPS Empress ceramic restorations in general practice. Int J Prosthodont 2003; 16:621–625.

Howden GF. Erosion as the presenting symptom in hiatus hernia. A case report. Br Dent J 1971; 131:455–456.

Iida K, Inokoshi S, Kurosaki N. Interfacial gaps following ceramic inlay cementation vs direct composites. Oper Dent 2003; 28:445–452.

Kakaboura A, Rahiotis C, Zinelis S, Al-Dhamadi YA, Silikas N, Watts DC. In vitro characterization of two laboratory-processed resin composites. Dent Mater 2003; 19:393–398.

Kelly PG, Smales RJ. Long-term cost-effectiveness of single indirect restorations in selected dental practices. Br Dent J 2004; 196:639–643.

Komine F, Tomic M, Gerds T, Strub JR. Influence of different adhesive resin cements on the fracture strength of aluminum oxide ceramic posterior crowns. J Prosthet Dent 2004; 92:359–364.

Lehmann F, Eickemeyer G, Rammelsberg P. Fracture resistance of metal-free composite crowns-effects of fiber reinforcement, thermal cycling, and cementation technique. J Prosthet Dent 2004; 92:258–264.

References

Manhart J, Mehl A, Obermeier T, Hickel R. Finite element study on stress distribution in dependence on cavity width and materials properties. Academy of Dental Materials: Proceedings of Conference on Clinically Appropriate Alternatives to Amalgam: Biophysical Factors in Restorative Decision-Making, October 30–November 2 1996; Munich, Germany, 9:269.

Martin N, Jedynakiewicz NM. Clinical performance of CEREC ceramic inlays: a systematic review. Dent Mater 1999; 15:54–61.

May KB, Russell MM, Razzoog ME, Lang BR. Precision of fit: the Procera AllCeram crown. J Prosthet Dent 1998; 80:394–404.

McClaren EA, White SN. Survival of In-Ceram crowns in a private practice: A prospective clinical trial. J Prosthet Dent 2000; 83:216–222.

Milosevic A, Agrawal N, Redfearn P, Mair L. The occurrence of toothwear in users of Ecstasy (3,4-methylenedioxymethamphetamine). Community Dent Oral Epidemiol 1999; 27:283–287.

Moazzez R, Bartlett D, Anggiansah A. Dental erosion, gastro-oesophageal reflux disease and saliva: how are they related? J Dent 2004; 32:489–494.

Molin MK, Karlsson SL. A randomized 5-year clinical evaluation of 3 ceramic inlay systems. Int J Prosthodont 2000; 13:194–200.

Nakamura T, Dei N, Kojima T, Wakabayashi K. Marginal and internal fit of Cerec 3 CAD/CAM all-ceramic crowns. Int J Prosthodont 2003; 16:244–248.

Oden A, Andersson M, Krystek-Ondracek I, Magnusson D. Five-year clinical evaluation of Procera AllCeram crowns. J Prosthet Dent 1998; 80:450–456.

Otto T, De Nisco S. Computer-aided direct ceramic restorations: a 10-year prospective clinical study of Cerec CAD/CAM inlays and onlays. Int J Prosthodont 2002; 15:122–128.

Owens BM, Halter TK, Brown DM. Microleakage of tooth-colored restorations with a beveled gingival margin. Quintessence Int 1998; 29:356–361.

Posselt A, Kerschbaum T. Longevity of 2,328 chairside Cerec inlays and onlays. Int J Comput Dent 2003; 6:231–248.

Reiss B. Klinische Langzeiterfahrungen mit Cerec-Inlays. Freie Zahnarzt 1994; 38:30–33.

Rosenstiel SF, Land MF, Rashid RG. Dentists' molar restoration choices and longevity: a web-based survey. J Prosthet Dent 2004; 91:363–367.

Sideridou I, Achilias DS, Kyrikou E. Thermal expansion characteristics of light-cured dental resins and resin composites. Biomaterials 2004; 25:3087–3097.

Sjogren G, Molin M, van Dijken JW. A 10-year prospective evaluation of CAD/CAM-manufactured (Cerec) ceramic inlays cemented with a chemically cured or dual-cured resin composite. Int J Prosthodont 2004; 17:241–246.

Sobrinho LC, Cattell MJ, Knowles JC. Fracture strength of all-ceramic crowns. J Mater Sci Mater Med 1998; 9:555–559.

Spohr AM, Sobrinho LC, Consani S, Sinhoreti MA, Knowles JC. Influence of surface conditions and silane agent on the bond of resin to IPS Empress 2 ceramic. Int J Prosthodont 2003; 16:277–282.

Thordrup M, Isidor F, Horsted-Bindslev P. A 5-year clinical study of indirect and direct resin composite and ceramic inlays. Quintessence Int 2001; 32:199–205.

Uno S, Finger WJ, Fritz UB. Effect of cavity design on microleakage of resin-modified glass ionomer restorations. Am J Dent 1997; 10:32–35.

van Dijken JW, Hasselrot L, Ormin A, Olofsson AL. Restorations with extensive dentin/enamel-bonded ceramic coverage. A 5-year follow-up. Eur J Oral Sci 2001; 109:222–229.

Walls AWG, Steele JG, Wassell RW. Crowns and other extra-coronal restorations: Porcelain laminate veneers. Br Dent J 2002; 193:73–82.

Young WG, Khan F. Sites of dental erosion are saliva-dependent. J Oral Rehabil 2002; 29:35–43.

Xu HC, Liu WY, Wang T. Measurement of thermal expansion coefficient of human teeth. Aust Dent J 1989; 34:530–535.

Subject Index

4-META resin   43, 44, 55, 116

acrylic splint   104
age   87
air abrasion   21
alumina   21
– as an abrasive   21, 103, 112
– as constituent of In-Ceram   115
– as constituent of Procera AllCeram   116
amalgam repair   36, 44, 60
amalgam repairing   37
amalgapins   43
amelogenesis imperfecta   84
articulating paper   56, 59, 71
articulator   70
atraumatic restorative treatment (ART)   24

Belleglass HP   106
bonded amalgam   43, 44
bulk fracture   35, 107, 108, 113
butt joint in indirect inlays/onlays   106

"C" factor   51
CAD/CAM   111, 118
calcium hydroxide   23, 38–41, 58, 87
caries-detector dyes   25
carisolv gel   23
cement lining   35
ceramic inserts   52
Cerec 3   111, 112
chlorhexidine   28–30
circumferential grooving   43
compomer   24, 100, 101

dental pulp   18, 19, 22, 24, 25, 38, 39, 42, 54, 78, 87, 88
dentinal sensitivity   99
DIAGNOdent   5–7, 12, 13
DIFOTI   7, 8, 13

emergence profile   76, 81
enamel demineralization   9, 10

feldspathic porcelain   85, 109, 112, 116
fissure sealants   55
flowable composite   58, 64
fluoride   33
– fluoride gel   29
– fluoride mouthwash   28, 29, 89
– fluoride varnish   29, 90
– glass ionomer   62, 102
– glass ionomer cements   73
– resin-modified glass ionomer   100
– Xeno III   103
FOTI   8

gingival inflammation   67
gingivitis   67

HEMA   55, 99, 100
hybrid layer   17, 55, 57

interproximal caries   8, 10, 11, 67

lasers   18
– erbium:YAG   18
– femtosecond laser   20
Lava ceramic   118
leucite-reinforced porcelain   85, 113

line angles of teeth   42, 76, 105

medical history   13, 27
microabrasion   90
microleakage   5, 39, 40, 43, 45, 54, 58, 73, 81, 82, 85, 100–102, 107, 117

nanocomposites   54
nanoleakage   55, 57

occlusal wear   34
occlusion   54, 56, 59, 60, 70, 79, 87, 98, 109, 112, 113
ozone therapy   32

photoactivated disinfection   23
polymerization shrinkage   51, 52, 54, 57, 58, 62, 64, 81, 101, 102, 105
postoperative sensitivity   83, 87, 89, 90
pulpal exposure   38–41
pulpal inflammation   19, 39, 40, 45, 90
pulpitis   38

quantitative light-induced fluorescence   9

radiographs   3, 10–13, 31
ramped light-curing units   52
resin modified glass ionomers   58, 62, 101, 115

restoration failure   26, 35
retention grooves   34, 57
retraction cord   77, 102, 117
root caries   33

saliva
– in caries risk   27, 30, 98
– in noncarious tooth wear   95
secondary caries   4, 5, 7, 10, 24, 26, 35–37, 43, 62, 102, 107, 113
self-etching primer   58, 59, 105
sensitivity   4–6, 8–10, 12, 45, 57
"shrink-free" resin composite   64
Sinfony   106
specificity   4, 6, 9, 10

Targis/Vectris   106
tenderness to percussion   38, 69
tertiary dentin   3, 40, 41
tooth fracture   37, 61, 112
"total etch" technique   54

Vitapan shade guide   75

walking bleach   88
white-spot lesion   1

xerostomia   4, 27

zinc oxide eugenol restorative material   39